HANDBOOK OF

community mental health

MEPC Handbook Series

- A. James Giannini, M.D., Henry R. Black, M.D., and Roger L. Goettsche, M.D.: *Psychiatric, Psychogenic, and Somatopsychic Disorders Handbook*
- Charles Toback, Ph.D.: *Pediatrician's Psychological Handbook*
- Donald G. Langsley, M.D., Irving N. Berlin, M.D., and Richard M. Yarvis, M.D., M.P.H.: *Handbook of Community Mental Health*

MEPC HANDBOOK SERIES

HANDBOOK OF

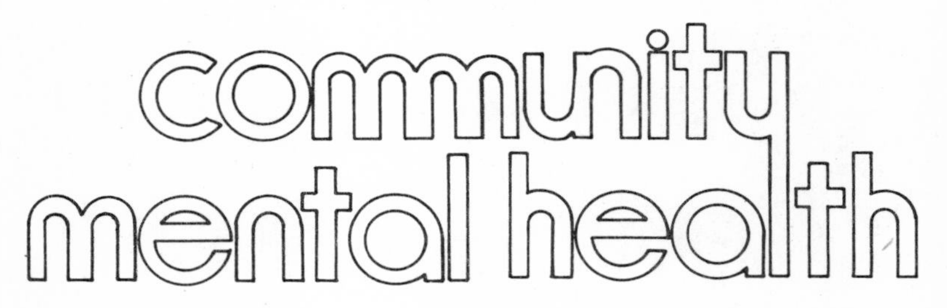

A PRACTICAL GUIDE TO THE OPERATION OF COMMUNITY MENTAL HEALTH CENTERS AND THE SERVICES THEY PROVIDE

DONALD G. LANGSLEY, M.D.
Professor of Psychiatry
University of Cincinnati College of Medicine

IRVING N. BERLIN, M.D.
Professor of Psychiatry
Director, Division of Child and Adolescent Psychiatry
Director, Children's Psychiatric Center
University of New Mexico School of Medicine

RICHARD M. YARVIS, M.D., M.P.H.
President, Pyramid Systems
Clinical Associate Professor of Psychiatry
University of California, Davis, School of Medicine

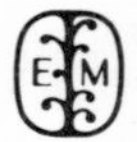
Medical Examination Publishing Co., Inc.
an Excerpta Medica company

Langsley, Donald G. (date)
Handbook of community mental health.

Bibliography: p.
Includes index.
1. Community mental health services — United States — Administration. I. Berlin, Irving, Norman (date). II. Yarvis, Richard M. III. Title. [DNLM: 1. Community mental health centers — Organization and administration — Handbooks. 2. Delivery of health care — Organization and administration — Handbooks. WM 30 L285h]
RA790.6.L37 362.2'2'0973 81-3933
ISBN 0-87488-605-8 AACR2

MEDICAL EXAMINATION PUBLISHING CO., INC.
an Excerpta Medica company
969 Stewart Avenue
Garden City, New York

August 1981

Printed in the United States of America

To Our Wives

Polly, Deane, and Phyllis

Introduction

This handbook is meant to be a practical guide to the operation of a community mental health center (CMHC) rather than a theoretical explanation of community mental health or of social psychiatry. It is designed to be of use to the psychiatrists, psychologists, social workers, nurses, and other mental health staff (including paraprofessionals and volunteers) who operate these programs of service to the mentally ill. Though recognizing that the community mental health approach has many aspects of a social movement, we are more concerned with health care service delivery than with social change, more involved with direct care than with primary prevention, and more committed to the quality and accessibility of care than to undoing social injustice.

We assume that a CMHC is defined by its commitment to a population. That population includes children, the aged, whole families, the underprivileged and those with chronic mental illness, as well as young adults with acute stress who seek psychotherapy to help overcome psychic blocks in achieving their potential. A CMHC is an institution which operates a variety of services designed to meet the needs of the many types of patients it serves. It uses a multidisciplinary mental health team with appropriate roles and activities not only for the psychiatrist and child psychiatrist, but for the social workers, nurses, psychologists and paraprofessionals on the staff as well. It is an institution which is part of the health care system, including state mental hospitals, and yet it also relates to social services and links with other human service agencies. It is committed to prevention, but recognizes the limits of primary prevention at this time and is generally more involved with secondary prevention. It is committed to ongoing program evaluation as one element in the planning process for new mental health services and rearrangement of existing services. It is involved with the community in defining mental health problems and in planning ways to solve those problems.

It is as true today as it was in 1963 when President John F. Kennedy said:

> Mental illness and mental retardation are among our most critical health problems. They occur more frequently, affect more people, require more prolonged treatment, cause more suffering by the families of the afflicted, waste more of our human resources and constitute more financial drain upon both the Public Treasury and the personal finances of the individual families than any other single condition....The time has come for a bold new approach.

New medical, scientific and social tools and insights are now available.

As a service delivery system, the CMHC is still in its adolescence. It is only 15 years since the federal government enacted legislation authorizing support for the staff and programs of such centers. Since 1965, over 700 CMHC's have been developed. They serve nearly half of the population of the United States. They have been instrumental in shifting the focus of the care of mental illness from state hospitals to the community. State hospital populations have dropped to a third of the numbers who were residents of such institutions 25 years ago. The development of the psychoactive medications and the new psycho-social treatment approaches (including the CMHC) has made it possible to treat most acute mental disorders in the community and to avoid unnecessary institutionalization for many. But this movement has not been without problems, some of them serious.

The most serious criticism of the CMHC has been the neglect of patients, especially the chronically mentally ill persons who used to be patients in state mental hospitals and were discharged to the community before programs were developed to meet their needs. CMHC's have been criticized when they give more attention to social issues (e.g., poverty and racism) than to the specific health care needs of those who live in the community. They have been criticized because many have developed an antimedical and even antiprofessional attitude which has discouraged the psychiatrists vitally needed as part of the mental health team from working in such centers. They have been charged with neglecting the needs of some populations, especially children, the aged, minorities and the chronically ill. They have suffered from a lack of financial support and from lack of adequate coverage of mental illness under insurance and other third-party payment for health care.

In spite of these criticisms, the CMHC offers more promise for treatment and prevention close to home than any existing or planned delivery system. After a year of study, the President's Commission on Mental Health affirmed the potential and usefulness of this system of care. It has previously been supported by the Congress and legislation is now in process to improve the programs, correct some of the deficiencies and arrange for the availability of services to all who need them.

We hope that this volume will be of some use to the tens of thousands of professionals and citizens involved in the CMHC's of this country.

Contents

notice

The editor(s) and/or author(s) and the publisher of this book have made every effort to ensure that all therapeutic modalities that are recommended are in accordance with accepted standards at the time of publication.

The drugs specified within this book may not have specific approval by the Food and Drug Administration in regard to the indications and dosages that are recommended by the editor(s) and/or author(s). The manufacturer's package insert is the best source of current prescribing information.

CHAPTER 1

HISTORY OF COMMUNITY MENTAL HEALTH

Donald G. Langsley, M.D.

1. The community mental health movement has its origin in concepts of:

   a) Treatment close to home rather than institutional care of psychiatric patients outside of the community

   b) Emphasis on prevention of illness rather than treatment after it has developed

   c) An eclectic approach to the use of all appropriate and useful treatment methods

   d) A commitment to meet the mental health needs of the total population rather than a responsibility for only those who come for treatment

   e) The traditional responsibility of government for the mentally ill in contrast to the responsibility of the individual and family for most physical illnesses

2. During the 18th and 19th centuries, care of the mentally ill was carried on in asylums or hospitals.

a) The mentally ill population consisted predominantly of poor people whose behavior was not controllable by family or community or those who had no families or social support.

b) The institutions were custody-oriented, designed more to protect society than to treat or cure. The inmates of such institutions were considered "alienated" from society. Psychiatrists of that era were called "alienists."

3. Psychiatric practice focused on the identification and classification of mental illness. Since there were few (if any) treatments, and since patients once committed (indefinitely) were expected to remain for years or for life, the role of the psychiatrist was one of classifier and warder, rather than healer. Most psychiatrists worked in such public-supported institutions. A few worked in private sanitaria or hospitals for the wealthy, or in medical schools where psychiatry had low status.

4. Psychiatric education used to consist of a few lectures demonstrating psychotic syndromes. It began in the 1870's, but even by 1909, the Council on Medical Education of the AMA recommended no more than a total of 30 hours of psychiatric education in the medical curriculum.

a) By 1940, psychiatric teaching occupied an average of 112 hours in the medical curriculum, and by 1966, the average was 458 hours.

b) Modern psychiatric education includes material on basic behavioral sciences as well as the commonly seen psychiatric syndromes and their treatment.

5. "Care" in public institutions for the mentally ill in the 18th and 19th centuries consisted of concern for basic needs (food, clothing and shelter) and physical health. Rehabilitation focused on discipline, manual labor, occupational-recreational activities and exhortative encouragement of thought control. Group meetings (including prayer) were common. Physical restraint was used to control unacceptable behavior. Institutions were small, usually with less than 200 patients.

a) In the second half of the 19th and first half of the 20th centuries (with the rise of urban population), the number of patients in such institutions increased dramatically and the institutions became overcrowded and understaffed. Physical control increased and the philosophy of moral treatment or rehabilitation of the individual disappeared.

6. Mental illness was then explained by heredity or as unspecified organic disease of the central nervous system.

   a) Two scientists helped change such views of mental illness:

      (1) Freud's discoveries of unconscious motivation and psychic determinism pointed to an etiologic explanation of mental illness and suggested therapy for at least some types of mental illness.

      (2) Adolf Meyer suggested that mental illness was a behavioral reaction to biological, psychological and social phenomena. Meyer also favored community based health centers where various human services could work with mental hospitals to promote early identification and treatment of mental illness. He also suggested community treatment after hospitalization. He proposed public education to promote mental health.

7. The <u>mental hygiene</u> movement emerged at the beginning of the 20th century. It was a citizen approach led by those who had been patients (or whose family members had been patients). It identified mental illness as a problem requiring public attention and government intervention. The National Association was founded in 1909.

   a) Clifford Beers' book <u>A Mind that Found Itself</u> (1905) was instrumental in getting public attention.

   b) Thomas Salmon developed screening and early treatment plans for the military around World War I, thus getting more attention focused on the problem of mental illness.

8. The <u>child guidance</u> movement (1920's) suggested that meeting the mental health needs of children would prevent adult psychopathology. This movement also introduced the concept of the interdisciplinary team for the treatment and prevention of mental illness.

9. Military psychiatry was one of the forerunners of community mental health.

   a) More attention was paid to screening psychiatric illness in draftees after the poor experience of World War I.

   b) Studies of war neuroses suggested insights into concepts of decompensation (crisis) in previously healthy individuals.

   c) Immediate treatment close to the front lines gave a high rate of return to duty. This suggested an approach that could apply to civilian models.

   d) Experience with hospitalization far behind the lines gave poorer results in rate of return to duty. Hospitalization at a distance seemed to promote chronicity.

   e) VA Hospitals were developed in nonurban areas. The VA also developed domiciliaries for the chronically dependent who did not require acute hospitalization. The experience between World Wars I and II suggested that these types of services promoted chronicity and encouraged institutionalism.

10. The mental hospital movement began with Dorothea Lynde Dix in the post-Civil War period. She led a citizen movement to provide humane care for the mentally ill.

    a) During the early to middle 20th century, mental hospitals became crowded and understaffed. Custody rather than treatment was the general approach.

    b) Hospitalization was assumed to be long-term - years to life.

    c) The hospitals were located away from urban centers, a fact which made it difficult for families to be involved in treatment and rehabilitation. Extrusion from the family was a common phenomenon.

    d) Studies of institutions made it clear that such approaches promoted dependency and chronicity.

    e) Studies of staff conflict and its effect on patient behavior contributed to the suggestion that the behavior of the chronic psychotic was as much a function of the treatment as the illness.

f) British hospitals demonstrated that doors could be unlocked and that a therapeutic milieu was an effective part of hospital treatment.

11. Somatic treatments for mental illness. A number of somatic treatments for psychiatric illness were developed during the 1930's. The result was to lend a certain therapeutic optimism to the mental hospital. The treatments developed included:

    a) Metrazol-induced convulsive therapy
    b) Electroconvulsive therapy
    c) Insulin coma therapy
    d) Indoklon convulsive therapy
    e) Prefrontal lobotomy

12. Crisis intervention. Leaning heavily on the experience of military psychiatry and disaster psychology, interest in crisis theory evolved from the work of Lindemann and Caplan.

    a) Crisis intervention demonstrated that acute decompensation represented an opportunity for either regression or growth.

    b) Crisis intervention contributed to the preventive-early intervention public health approach which was to characterize community mental health.

13. Psychoactive drugs. Antipsychotic, antidepressant and antianxiety drugs have markedly altered the practice of psychiatry.

    a) Early experiments demonstrated the antipsychotic properties of rauwolfia alkaloids. This was followed by the introduction of chlorpromazine, which since the early 1950's has been the most frequently used antipsychotic drug.

    b) Antidepressants emerged from the use of mono-amine oxidase inhibitors in the treatment of tuberculosis. Serious side effects and the need for more predictable therapeutic results caused a shift to tricyclics.

    c) Anti-anxiety drugs have become the most frequently prescribed medications in the pharmacopeia. A plethora of various types have evolved. The demand for financial rewards has spurred pharmaceutical companies to develop a large number of anti-anxiety drugs.

d) The antipsychotic and antidepressant medications have permitted many patients to be treated outside hospitals and have reduced the use of ECT, insulin coma therapy, and other drastic somatic therapies, as well as prefrontal lobotomy.

e) Interest in biologic models of mental illness was spurred by the psychoactive drugs. The relation of target behavior to specific drugs suggested biochemical approaches to understanding human behavior.

14. Alternatives to hospitalization. The development of pharmacotherapy and the increasing use of psychiatric wards in general hospitals encouraged those who felt that patients with serious mental illness could be treated outside a mental hospital. A variety of techniques were reported during the 1950's and 1960's. They include:

a) Crisis intervention. Twenty-four-hour immediate aid by telephone or in person. These units are usually staffed by mental health professionals, though some operate with volunteers or paraprofessionals with professional backup. They may be located in the emergency rooms of general hospitals or may be administratively and physically separate. The goal of these centers is to deal with acute and immediate problems through immediate evaluation and brief outpatient treatment. Evaluation studies have shown that this type of service can prevent hospitalization. It is a service that may be family- or individual-oriented.

b) Telephone hotlines are often included in the immediate treatment-crisis intervention services. They may be oriented to the suicide (Suicide Prevention Centers) or to specialized groups (adolescents, drug users, etc). As a referral unit, they are often most frequently used to obtain information and referral.

c) Half-way houses. Various alternatives to twenty-four-hour hospitalization include half-way houses or alternative residential arrangements. They have been used to provide supervised living for those who are suffering acute decompensation (half-way-in) or as a transitional setting for those who have been hospitalized and require supervised arrangements before achieving independent living. They may be operated directly by community mental health centers (CMHC's) or by community agencies with CMHC consultation. There should be some training of the residential center staff (non-professionals, usually) and access to the CMHC resources.

d) Other residential care. Other models of residential care have been developed, including Board and Care Homes. The size varies (from no more than six patients in California to up to one hundred in certain settings on the East Coast). The training and backup services offered by a CMHC are essential elements. Those which have been small and closely associated with a total and comprehensive CMHC program have probably been the most successful. A large portion of the population of such settings are patients who have previously been in a state mental hospital.

e) Partial hospitalization. Day hospital, night hospital, weekend hospital and various combinations have been developed, but the day hospital has been the most frequently tested and used model. Patients who would ordinarily be hospitalized in a 24-hour unit may be involved in a five day per week, eight hours per day program. The goal is to continue to have the patient live at home and to maintain the family relationships which will offer support for ongoing living arrangements. The program has been especially useful for the chronically mentally ill, though it has been used for acute illness as well. The Fort Logan (Denver, Colorado) experience has shown that at least 70% of those who used to be hospitalized in a 24-hour unit can be treated in this manner. The treatment program includes all of the services and programs found in a 24-hour unit.

f) Outpatient therapy. An outpatient service receives referral from crisis services which have treated the acutely ill patient to the point of recompensation, but where the patient now requires more long-term or reconstructive therapy. Outpatient clinics also include such programs as medication-aftercare clinics. Outpatient treatment with supportive psychotherapy and medication has been shown to prevent hospitalization as well as to serve as an alternative.

15. Legislation associated with community mental health. The community mental health movement has been associated with professional and government leadership. The laws and steps involved include:

a) 1946 National Health Act provided for the education of mental health professionals. It recognized the short supply and its success should be noted by the increase of psychiatrists (from 5,000 in 1946 to 30,000 in 1979) as well as by similar increases of professionals in clinical psychology, psychiatric social work and psychiatric nursing.

b) 1949 - Establishment of NIMH. The National Institute of Mental Health was established in 1949 with a tripartite mission of supporting education, research and service. The service responsibilities made it different from the other National Institutes of Health. Later reorganizations have created a separate (and higher level) organization called Alcoholism, Drug Abuse and Mental Health Administration (ADAMHA). In part this was a response to the alcoholism and drug abuse groups who did not want to be "under mental health".

c) 1955-61 Joint Commission on Mental Health and Illness. With professional leadership and the support of Dr. Robert Felix (first Director of NIMH), a 1955 law created a Commission on Mental Health and Mental Illness. The basic publication, Action for Mental Health, appeared in 1961 and was the major proposal for a community mental health movement.

d) 1963 Community Mental Health Center Act. A message by President Kennedy prompted the passage of the 1963 CMHC Act, the first legislation propounding the basic structure of CMHC's. It provided mostly for construction funds, but established the basic definitions (size of catchment area, concept of comprehensive services, certain required services) and got the federal government firmly into the business of supporting direct and preventive mental health services. It also established the principles of continuity of care and of community/consumer participation in community mental health services planning and program implementation.

e) 1965 CMHC Staffing Act. The 1965 legislation provided for federal subsidy of staffing costs. There was to be a gradual reduction in federal share and an increase in community share. The act was an extension of the federal construction support in 1963 legislation.

f) 1970 Amendments to the CMHC Act. In 1970, certain amendments to the 1965 legislation provided special grants for child mental health programs, drug abuse programs and alcoholism programs. There were also special provisions for increasing federal share and extending the period of the grants in poverty areas.

g) 1975 - P.L. 93-64. In the 1975 legislation, the Congress affirmed the interest of the federal government in providing mental health services and acknowledged the usefulness of the community mental health movement. Certain technical redefinitions of community mental health centers occurred, but the basic philosophy was continued and extended.

h) President's Commission on Mental Health. In 1977, President Jimmy Carter appointed a Commission on Mental Health chaired by his wife Rosalynn. That group recommended certain "mid-course corrections" but retained the Community Mental Health approach as a basic structure for mental health care. They also recommended the passage of a Mental Health Systems Act which was accomplished in 1980.

16. Effects of the community mental health movement. By 1977, the community mental health movement had had a profound effect on the broad area of mental health and mental illness. It has been called the fourth psychiatric revolution (the others being freeing so-called mental prisoners from chains, the discovery of the unconscious and opening the locked wards of mental hospitals). Without doubt, treatment in the community would not have been possible without the discovery of the antipsychotic and antidepressant medications, or without some of the coexistent social changes which began to alter the concept of the mentally ill from one of stigmatization to one of a treatable illness. Some of the effects of the community mental health movement might be listed as follows:

a) Establishment of CMHC's. As of 1979, over 700 federally funded centers have been operational. This does not include many other CMHC's that have not necessarily received federal support. In California, all 58 counties have a publicly funded mental health program with at least the five basic services (emergency service, inpatient, partial hospitalization, outpatient and consultation-education services). New York, Michigan, Illinois, Massachusetts and others have been leaders and have more or less successfully provided such mental health services to large populations. It is estimated that more than 60% of the total U.S. population is within reasonable travel distance from a CMHC.

b) Reduced use of state hospitals. Both resident patient populations and numbers of admissions to state mental hospitals have declined dramatically. Over the past ten years in California, state hospital populations have dropped from 36,000 to less than 5,000. In Sacramento County, California (population 700,000) admissions per year dropped from 1200 to 35. Although these may not be representative of the whole country, the trend is apparent. In California, five state mental hospitals have closed or have terminated their programs for the mentally ill or have concentrated their services on the developmentally disabled (mentally retarded).

c) Increased mental health manpower. There have been marked expansions in numbers in each of the mental health professions as well as major changes in the role of each of the professions. Psychiatrists, for example, have increased from 5,000 in the mid 1940's to 30,000. Clinical psychology was "born" after World War II and has grown tremendously. The same is true of mental health nursing and social work. Roles for each profession have expanded - some class it as "role blurring", but it is quite apparent that there are areas of overlapping skills as well as distinctive roles and competences. In nursing and social work, professional education levels have risen to make the Master's Degree the expected level of formal credentials - more in social work than nursing. There have also been struggles between the professions - especially over the right to do solo private practice. Paraprofessionals or new professions have been developed and found to have a useful purpose in a community mental health center. As with all changes, the pendulum swings, and in some areas there has developed an anti-professionalism and anti-intellectualism along with a move toward more community control and less power and decision making for professional groups.

d) New problems, new populations. A definition of the proper concerns for mental health groups has been extended to cover new target populations and additional problems. For the most part, these new problems reflect a traditional "illness model" and the recognition of the important role of social forces and political problems. These new problems have included:

(1) Children who have generally been the most underserved group.

(2) Drug abuse, a broad spectrum of problems obviously influenced by poverty, urban problems, and the alienation of younger people from adult generations.

(3) Alcoholism, long a serious problem but now recognized as not simply criminal behavior. Though the criminal justice forces have done little except to use "drunk tanks", it must also be admitted that traditional mental health resources have shown little success in dealing with this problem.

(4) The aged. With life expectation increasing, there are more and more "senior citizens" in the community. Many of their problems have been shown to be treatable and the wholesale warehousing of such individuals has been changed.

(5) Minority and poverty populations. Traditionally, these groups have been underserved by mental health programs. The community mental health movement has moved to include such populations in planning appropriate services and to better meet their needs.

e) Involvement of the judiciary. In the past, the legislatures have been the moving forces in changing social services and in producing new programs. More recently, the judiciary has taken a leading role. Class action suits and a willingness of many courts to make new laws have resulted in decisions such as the right to treatment, new definitions of confidentiality and greater attention to civil rights and due process.

f) Community control, community participation. The community mental health movement has emphasized the involvement of populations served in the planning process. The partnership between community and professionals has made many decisions more relevant, but it has also endured certain strains. There have been some in the community who feel that even decisions traditionally made by professionals should be subject to community review. Others have felt that the funds (and jobs) put into mental health services could be used to create jobs for unemployed minorities. There are a number of models of CMHC's going all the way from direct governmental control and hiring of all staff (with citizen advisory boards) to community boards hiring the professionals and receiving government and other third party funds.

g) Other concerns and criticisms have included:

(1) Lack of special programs and adequate attention to the chronically ill (mostly former state hospital patients).

(2) Dangerous patients are discharged from the hospital and loosened on the community.

(3) The catchment area concept is unwieldy and unrealistic for most rural and many urban communities.

(4) Services in rural areas are sadly lacking and and poorly adapted to the special needs imposed by geography and thinly populated areas.

(5) Services to children and to minority and poverty populations are inadequate and inappropriate.

(6) There is a very visible anti-mental health movement which uses certain civil rights and issues of governmental control to attack the mental health movement.

CHAPTER 2

DEFINITION OF COMMUNITY MENTAL HEALTH

Richard M. Yarvis, M.D., M.P.H.

1. Introduction: This chapter will develop a definition of community mental health in three sections:

    a) The presentation of several models which define community mental health

    b) A discussion of some issues which are relevant to any definition of community mental health

    c) A definition which draws upon the insights presented in a) and b)

2. Some models which define community mental health include:

    a) The National Institute of Mental Health Model: This model was originally articulated in P.L. 88-164 and P.L. 94-63, the original and the most recent pieces of federal community mental health legislation. The model has been further articulated in regulations set down by the NIMH and consists of the following characteristics:

(1) Mental health services for a given geographical area (catchment area) should be the responsibility of a community mental health center (CMHC).

(2) The size of catchment areas should be determined by population density and optimally should include 125-150,000 residents.

(3) A comprehensive range of services should be offered by each center which must include "five essential services": inpatient, partial hospitalization, outpatient, crisis-emergency and consultation and education.

These original five essential services were expanded in 1975 to include specialized services for children and for the aged, screening for potential state hospital cases and follow-up for state hospital admissions, a half-way house, services for drug abusers and alcoholics and a program evaluation effort.

(4) Centers should provide continuity of care to patients so that services will not be fragmented. The expectation here was for patients to obtain all needed mental health services from a single source.

(5) All possible attempts should be made to render care to patients within their own communities. The use of facilities outside the catchment area such as state hospitals should be kept at the lowest feasible level.

b) The Public Health Model: This model has been articulated by such pioneers in CMH as Duhl,[1] Caplan,[2] Lemkau,[3] and Bellak[4] and is organized within the framework of three basic public health principles:

(1) Primary prevention. Community mental health programs must focus on health promotion and on specific protection in order to prevent the occurrence of mental illness. As such, they will develop programs which focus on such areas as child-rearing, adequate mothering and the attainment of developmental benchmarks. Programs will also focus on specific protection (e.g., aid in preparation for surgery or some other traumatic event).

(2) Secondary prevention. Community mental health programs must focus on the early detection and rapid treatment of mental illness. Programs should develop screening techniques and an adequate range of mental health treatment programs.

(3) Tertiary prevention. Community mental health programs must focus on limiting permanent disability from mental illness and on reversing as much damage as possible. The CMHC should develop programs to reverse regression, eliminate dysfunctional symptomatology and improve adaptations to community life.

c) The Social Activist Model: This model has been articulated by Duhl[5] and Riessman[6] and by Peck, Kaplan and Roman[7] among others. It is organized around a number of basic concepts:

(1) Mental illness cannot be viewed in isolation from the social and economic conditions in which it occurs but must be viewed as one end product of the interplay of social and economic forces on the individual.

(2) Community mental health programs must encourage and aid social action programs whose aim is to improve the lot of persons living in the community.

(3) Social action components should be built into community mental health programs by recruiting community organizers to develop the abilities of indigenous community groups to obtain better housing, recreation, employment and education.

(4) Community mental health programs should act as an agent to break down the barriers between other public service agencies and their constituents. This could mean becoming actively involved in the political process.

(5) Center services should be as close to the community they serve as possible.

(6) Centers should emphasize small group interactions for both diagnosis and treatment and for social action interventions in the community as well.

(7) Centers should employ paraprofessionals who are trained by center personnel staff and who are indigenous to the community served. Such indigenous personnel often relate better to their communities, especially disadvantaged communities, than do the largely white and middle class professionals. They can, therefore, serve as a bridge between the professionals and the community. This does not eliminate the need for quality professional staff.

3. Pertinent issues which are relevant to any definition of community mental health include:

a) The suggestion has been offered that community mental health can be defined as a social institution set up to control and/or eradicate divergent political viewpoints. Persons offering this suggestion point to the Soviet Union where mental health facilities serve as places to correct "political deviance."

b) Kenniston[8] has examined this view and has found the evidence for it wanting. He has acknowledged that the potential for such practice exists. The authors agree with Kenniston's appraisal and point out that, if anything, some centers have served the opposite role.

c) A measure of "community control" has been considered by some as an integral part of the definition of community mental health.

(1) Community control means the delineation of community mental health program policies by a board made up of persons indigenous to the community in which the program operates and selected in such a way that they are representative of that community.

(2) Hobbs and Smith[9] contend that a community mental health center cannot be an effective agency without "community control."

(3) On occasion, this definition has led to significant conflict within centers which polarize staff and to conflict between centers and the politically active groups that operate within their

communities. Kaplan[10] has described one instance of this at Lincoln Hospital Mental Health Service in New York City.

d) A definition of community is a necessity if the "community" in community mental health is to be understood fully. Alternative conceptualizations of this term have been compiled by Register.[11] Using his scheme, the concept of community can be defined as:

(1) A geographical area - here the community includes all persons living within specified geographical boundaries.

(2) A majority - here the community is broadly defined to consist of the largest possible number of recipients within a given geographical area.

(3) A vocal minority - here the community is defined as a particular group which clamors with particular effectiveness for services or which has and exercises exceptional political clout to obtain services.

(4) Society at large - the most inclusive definition possible wherein all humanity is an eligible recipient for service.

(5) A categorical group - all members of the community share some common characteristic such as economic status, political affiliation, occupational role, union membership and so on.

(6) A group defined by a set of common beliefs - all members of the community share in some common philosophy or particular belief system.

(7) A group defined by some elitist concept - all members of the community have been chosen by the staff as being deserving of services. Such decisions may be intentional or subtle and not readily recognized by staff.

(8) Participants in some set of mutual interactions - all members of the community are participants in a set of interactions. All others are outsiders and are not eligible for services.

4. Ecology, a branch of inquiry devoted to attempts to better understand the nature of the interaction of human beings with their environment, has added yet another dimension to the definition of community mental health. According to Clausen and Kohn,[12] the important concerns of any community mental health program must include:

   a) The interactions of persons with their physical environment. Issues such as population density, the quality of public housing, the availability of recreational facilities are included.

   b) The interactions of persons with their social environment. Here the effects of the social matrix in which people live or their behavior must be considered.

   c) The interactions between a community mental health program and other social agencies in the community. The effects of the presence of each on the performance of the other must be explored.

5. The distinctions between community psychiatry and social psychiatry must be drawn in order to bring the definition of community mental health into sharp relief. Viola Bernard[13] has drawn this distinction with clarity. Drawing upon her and others, we suggest that:

   a) Social psychiatry focuses primarily on theory and develops concepts and hypotheses which are related to the interplay between the individual and the social systems, cultural matrices and physical environment which impact upon him.

   b) Community psychiatry (a term which we are using interchangeably with community mental health) focuses primarily on applied practice at the community level. The emphasis is on service programs and on evaluation of such programs.

   c) The concepts and hypotheses of social psychiatry will be modified as a consequence of discoveries at the applied level. Conversely, concepts and hypotheses from social psychiatry will shape the nature of applied programs which are developed at the community level.

6. Contrasts and conflicts between an "intrapsychic" and a "socio-cultural" model for understanding behavior and as

a basis for conceptualizing treatment interventions have been associated with community mental health.

a) Community mental health psychiatrists have been accused of failing to give sufficient weight to the intrapsychic dimension of human behavior. Conversely, some community-oriented psychiatrists have accused their psychoanalytically oriented colleagues of failing to give adequate attention to those social and cultural dimensions which influence behavior.

b) Any complete conceptualization of community mental health must include adequate attention to both the intrapsychic and the socio-cultural dimensions of human behavior.

7. Contrasts have been drawn between the mental hygiene clinic or outpatient psychiatric clinic on the one hand and the community mental health center on the other. Enumeration of several of the differences should help to highlight some of the key concepts that define community mental health.

a) The outpatient or mental hygiene clinic focuses on those patients who apply to it for treatment. It does not concern itself with any broader constituency. The community mental health center focuses on all of the persons that comprise its community. This will include patients who apply for treatment, impaired persons who do not apply (and hence need to be encouraged to) and healthy persons (at whom prevention efforts may be directed).

b) The outpatient or mental hygiene clinic generally offers a limited range of services. Patients requiring inpatient or partial hospitalization services, for instance, may have to be referred to a different service provider. Children may or may not be served. Crisis services may or may not be available. Prevention programs are not usually offered. The community mental health center usually provides a complete range of services both to adults and to children. Patients, therefore, do not have to be transferred to other service providers with the consequent loss of continuity of care. Prevention efforts as well as treatment are provided.

8. Community mental health has come to be defined, in part, by its application of particular intervention techniques which either have been pioneered in or have come into widespread use in community health centers. These include crisis intervention and the widespread use of time-limited treatment techniques. Also included are partial hospitalization (both the day and night hospital) and the use of the half-way house. Numerous preventive strategies including early childhood intervention projects, projects involving community education, consultation efforts with all kinds of social agencies and with schools have all flowered in connection with community mental health programs.

9. Another basic issue which has become identified with community mental health relates to the location where treatment takes place.

   a) An earlier model for rendering mental health services relied heavily on large state or county hospitals which were frequently located at some distance from the patient's home, family and friends.

   b) A prominent objective of community mental health is to treat all patients as close to home, family and friends as is feasible. Treatment facilities are located within the community. Satellite clinics bring the front line of treatment even closer to the patient's doorstep. Mobile crisis teams bring treatment right into the patient's own home. Center staff get out into the community regularly to work with schools, police, social agencies and the like. Various kinds of outreach programs attempt to encourage more community residents to make use of center resources.

10. A comprehensive model definition of community mental health will now be outlined below. It will draw upon much that has been presented above. Community mental health has the following characteristics:

    a) It is an organized set of <u>treatment, consultation, educational and preventive programs</u> directed at actual and potential mental health problems in a community.

    b) Its <u>objectives are the reduction of and prevention of mental illness</u> through <u>prevention</u> efforts, <u>early detection</u> programs and adequate <u>treatment</u> programs.

c) It accepts responsibility for the mental health needs of all persons residing in a community which has been defined by a set of geographical boundaries (a catchment area) or by membership in some categorical group (e.g., all members of a labor union). All members of the defined community are of active concern to the program, not just those patients who come for treatment.

d) It seeks to provide a comprehensive range of services which include all appropriate and necessary treatment services (inpatient, outpatient, partial hospitalization, crisis intervention) as well as all necessary consultation and education programs for community groups and social agencies.

e) It accepts as a prime objective the establishment and maintenance of continuity of care to each recipient of services. Services are designed to avoid fragmented and disjointed care.

f) It insists upon an adequate and ongoing planning effort which relies heavily upon assessments of community mental health needs. The needs assessment data is then used to design programs and to assign priorities for resource allocation. Resource allocation is related to need rather than to idiosyncratic staff interest. Changes in need are monitored and planning altered and resources reassigned accordingly.

g) It requires an active and continuous evaluation process in order to determine the efficiency, effectiveness, adequacy and appropriateness of all programs. Such evaluation data are then utilized in the planning and resource allocation process.

h) It seeks out and utilizes grass roots input from the residents of the community which it serves. This is accomplished by advisory boards, community forums and by active attention to and investigation of an active program which assesses patient satisfaction with service rendered. It may utilize community surveys to determine the views of community members. Under some circumstances, community members may share policy-making responsibility with program managers.

i) It attempts to maximize the extent to which services are rendered to patients within the community and to reduce the extent to which treatment resources outside the community must be used. Reduction of state hospital utilization and the reintegration of state hospital patients into the community are prime objectives of community mental health.

j) It directs special attention to those population groups within the community who are at special risk to mental illness (e.g., the poor, the unemployed, victims of traumatic events, those who have suffered loss) or who have been neglected and underserved (e.g., children, the elderly, minorities). This may require the development of special programs for such groups and/or special efforts to encourage them to utilize services.

k) It employs a strategy of active outreach efforts to increase the utilization of its services. Such efforts may include the use of techniques to improve public awareness of services and the use of public education programs to improve the community's understanding of mental health issues. It may include the use of satellite clinics and mobile clinics to improve the accessibility of services. It may include the use of mental health workers indigenous to the community being served who work to encourage community members to utilize services.

l) It utilizes a wide range of professionals and paraprofessionals to render all of its services to patients and to the community. Staff are utilized according to training and skill levels rather than on the basis of professional label. The recognition that mental health manpower resources are scarce leads to strong emphasis on inservice training.

REFERENCES

1. Duhl, L. The Psychiatric Evolution. In Concepts of Community Psychiatry. S. Goldston (Ed.). Bethesda: National Institute of Mental Health, 1965.

2. Caplan G. An Approach to Community Mental Health. New York: Grune and Stratton, 1966.

3. Lemkau, P. Prevention in Psychiatry. Am. J. Public Hlth. 55:554-560, 1965.

4. Bellak, L. Community Mental Health as a Branch of Public Health. In Progress in Community Mental Health. L. Bellak (Ed.). New York: Grune and Stratton, 1969.

5. Duhl, L. See Reference 1.

6. Riessman, F. and Miller, S. Social Change versus the "Psychiatric World View". Am. J. Orthopsychiatry 34:29-38, 1964.

7. Peck, H., Kaplan, S. and Roman, M. Prevention, Treatment and Social Action: A Strategy of Intervention in a Disadvantaged Urban Area. Am. J. Orthopsychiatry 36:57-69, 1966.

8. Kenniston, K. How Community Mental Health Stamped Out the Riots (1968-78). Transaction, July/August, 1968.

9. Smith, M. and Hobbs, M. The Community and the Community Mental Health Center. American Psychological Association, Washington, DC, 1966.

10. Kaplan, S. and Roman, M. The Organization and Delivery of Mental Health Services in the Ghetto. New York: Praeger, 1973.

11. Register, D. Community Mental Health - For Whose Community. Am. J. Public Hlth. 64:886-893, 1974.

12. Clausen, J. and Kohn, M. The Ecological Approach in Social Psychiatry. American Journal of Sociology 60: 140-151, 1954.

13. Bernard, V. Education for Community Psychiatry in a University Medical Center. In Handbook of Community Psychiatry and Community Mental Health. L. Bellak (Ed.). New York: Grune and Stratton, 1964.

14. Bloom, B. The Medical Model, Miasma Theory and Community Mental Health. Comm. Mental Hlth. J. 1:333-338, 1965.

15. Sabshin, M. Theoretical Models in Community and Social Psychiatry. In Community Psychiatry. Ed. L. Roberts. Madison: University of Wisconsin Press, 1966.

CHAPTER 3

THE USE OF EPIDEMIOLOGY IN MENTAL HEALTH PLANNING

Richard M. Yarvis, M.D., M.P.H.

1. Several kinds of epidemiological data are useful for planning mental health programs:

    a) Prevalence rates which measure overall impairment for a whole population, i.e., How many persons are currently impaired?

    b) Prevalence rates of impairment for specific demographic, social and economic groups within a given population, i.e., What is the age, sex, race, marital status, educational and income distribution of persons who are impaired?

    c) Incidence rates which measure the rate at which new cases of impairment arise in a given population, i.e., How many previously healthy persons have become impaired this year?

    d) Incidence rates for specific demographic, social and economic groups within a given population, i.e., Are healthy persons in one age, sex, race, marital status, educational or income group more likely to become impaired than healthy persons in another such group?

2. To be useful, epidemiological data should meet certain criteria:

    a) What constitutes "impairment" should be defined precisely.

    b) The methods used to determine which persons qualify as "impaired" should be accurate and reliable.

    c) The methods used to determine which persons qualify as "impaired" should be easily replicable from investigator to investigator.

3. Several terms are frequently used in the epidemiological literature and hence deserve definition:

    a) Epidemiology. This term refers to the study of the frequency and distribution of pathological conditions in a given population. Epidemiologists ask questions like: How many persons are ill or impaired? At what rate do new "cases" arise?

    b) Prevalence. The term refers to the number of active "cases" which are present in a given population at a single point or over a given period of time. Prevalence is usually expressed as the number of existing cases/per unit of population, e.g., 50 cases/100,000 population.

    c) Incidence. This term refers to the rate at which new "cases" appear in a given population over a defined period of time (frequently one year). Incidence is expressed as the number of new cases/per unit of population per year, e.g., 5 cases/100,000 population/year.

    d) A "case". This term refers to each individual who has some condition that the epidemiologist is interested in. In mental health work, "case" is defined as an individual who by virtue of mental illness has an impairment of normal expectable life functions and/or the manifestations of one or more symptoms of mental illness.

    e) Sensitivity. This term refers to the success with which a measuring instrument used to identify "cases" can identify them. A perfectly sensitive measuring instrument would identify every impaired individual in a population.

f) Specificity. This term refers to the success with which a measuring instrument does not misidentify a healthy individual as impaired. A perfectly specific measuring instrument would not identify any healthy individual as impaired.

4. None of the epidemiological data collected to date meet all of these criteria completely; in spite of this, some of the available data are worth applying to the planning process.

5. The available sources of mental health epidemiological data fall into several categories which have been defined according to how the data were collected. All involve prevalence data only.

   a) True epidemiological studies in which a whole population is sampled and diagnoses or estimates of impairment are made on the basis of clinical data. The two best examples of this type of study are summarized below.

      (1) In a study conducted in New York City in the late 1950's, the "Midtown Manhattan Study" (Srole et al., 1962),[1] a discrete geographic area with a population of 110,000 was selected.

         (a) Using survey sampling techniques, a sample of 1911 persons was selected to be interviewed. The sample included only adults between the ages of 20 and 59. The sample accurately reflected the actual age and sex distribution of the whole population in the 20-59 age group.

         (b) Of the 1911 individuals selected, 1660 persons agreed to be interviewed (an 87% interview completion rate).

         (c) Interviews were conducted using a questionnaire containing more than 200 items. This included data on demographic, social and economic characteristics, psychopathological signs and symptoms, social and occupational functioning, health status and psychiatric treatment.

(d) Once collected, the data for each respondent were analyzed independently by two psychiatrists and an impairment status was assigned. Each individual fell into one of six categories (well, mild impairment, moderate impairment, marked impairment, severe impairment, incapacitated).

(e) Some relevant findings from this study are cited in Table 1.

TABLE 1

MIDTOWN MANHATTAN STUDY

Well	18.5%
Mild symptom formation	36.3%
Moderate symptom formation	21.8%
Marked symptom formation	13.2%
Severe symptom formation	7.5%
Incapacitated	2.7%
Total impaired	23.4%

(2) In a study conducted in Canada, the "Stirling County Study" (D. Leighton et al., 1963),[2] a rural county in Nova Scotia with a population of 20,000 persons was selected.

(a) Using survey sampling techniques, a random sample, 1010 individuals, was chosen representing all adults aged 20 and older. The sample was found to be representative of the adult population.

(b) Using a questionnaire of more than 200 items, data were collected on demographic, social and economic characteristics, health, psychopathological signs and symptoms, childhood history and social and occupational functioning.

(c) Once collected, the data for each respondent were analyzed independently by two psychiatrists and impairment ratings assigned.

(d) Some relevant findings from this study are presented in Table 2.

TABLE 2

STIRLING COUNTY STUDY

Type V Probably well	17.4%
Type IV Doubtful	25.5%
Type III Probable disorder	37.1%
Type II Disorder with significant impairment	16.8%
Type I Most abnormal	3.2%
Total impaired (Type I and Type II)	20.0%

b) True epidemiological studies in which a whole population is sampled and estimates of impairment are made <u>on the basis of some standardized screening instrument</u>.

(1) A screening instrument. This is a written questionnaire that is designed to measure impairment levels, and hence to determine <u>who is a case</u>. One such instrument, the Langner Screening Scale, will be discussed later. The questionnaire provides a numerical score for each respondent. That score rates that respondent as being either healthy or impaired. The Langner Screening Scale was chosen for discussion here because it has been validated using clinical data.

(2) Screening instruments are useful because they enable investigators to examine large populations without large expenditures of resources. However, they have not proven to

be as accurate as studies based on clinical data primarily because of imperfections in the screening instruments themselves.

(3) Data from five studies conducted with adults in different locations are summarized in Table 3. All used the Langner Screening Scale which was developed originally in the Midtown Manhattan Study.

(4) Note that the rates in Table 3 are all lower than those cited in the Midtown and Stirling County Studies. Screening scales have been found to be quite specific but not very sensitive and thus to under-report the number of persons who are actually impaired.

(5) The Langner Screening Scale (Langner, 1962)[3] consists of 22 items, all of which were included originally in the Midtown Manhattan questionnaire.

The scale can either be administered by an interviewer or can be self-administered. It is not sensitive in picking up conditions like mental retardation, sociopathy or organic brain syndromes. It does not classify respondents by type of disorder. The scale is not time specific in its inquiry. The scale is quite specific but not very sensitive. Hence, false-positive results are rare but false-negative results are common.

c) The reader is directed to other epidemiological studies that have been done in the United States over the years. Space does not permit a thoroughgoing review of such studies but some overall findings from three of them will be cited later.

(1) Pasamanick,[8] in a study done in Baltimore, utilized data collected by nonpsychiatric physicians from a community sample and recorded an illness rate of 10.9%. It should be noted, however, that the records of one-third of the sample were not sufficiently complete to determine the presence or absence of mental illness.

TABLE 3

STUDIES USING LANGNER SCREENING SCALE

Study Site and Year	Sample, Size and Age Range	Sampling Process	% of Population with Significant Impairment
New York City, New York 1953 (Langner, 1962)[3]	1660 persons 20-59 years of age	Random sampling of households	11.2
Kalamazoo, Michigan 1959 (Manis, 1963 and 1964)[4]	1183 persons 20-59 years of age	Random sampling of households	12.0
Early, New Hampshire 1960's (Phillips, 1966)[5]	600 persons 20-59 years of age	Random sampling of households	8.7
Three communities in Nebraska, mid-1960's (Meilie, 1972)[6]	6016 persons 20 years or older	Random sampling of households	10.9
Houston, Texas 1969 (Gaitz and Scott, 1972)[7]	1441 persons 20 years or older	Nonrandom stratified sample selection for age, sex, ethnicity and occupation	14.5

(2) Cole and his co-workers[9] did a clinical study of a small community sample of respondents in Salt Lake City. He reported an illness rate of 32.0% in this population.

(3) Tischler and Myers and their co-workers[10] in a more recent ongoing study in New Haven have reported an impairment rate of 18.0%. Their study of a community sample utilizes a screening scale which was developed out of the Stirling County Study.

d) Epidemiological data for children are much more sparse than that for adults; still, some data are available and are worth discussion.

(1) In one recent study, Langner (the developer of the Langner Screening Scale) and co-workers[11] developed a screening instrument better suited to the assessment of children. While still in the developmental phase, it has already been tested in a study population of 1034 children, aged 6-18. The study was divided into two parts. The first part attempted to assess impairment using a 654-item questionnaire which was scored by psychiatrists and by computer analysis. This work yielded an overall impairment rate of 11.5%. The second part of the study experimented with a 35-question screening instrument which yielded an impairment rate of 14.5%. The screening instrument when calibrated against the first part of the study had a false-positive rate of 8.2% and a false-negative rate of 32.8%.

(2) Michael Shepherd and colleagues[12] working in England have measured levels of "deviance" in children based upon behavior and symptomatology such as bedwetting, truancy, nightmares, destructiveness, stealing and lying. This group uses a method which takes account of the number of symptoms or behaviors, the age of the child and the commonplaceness of the symptom or behavior at a given age as measured in a larger number of children. "Deviant" children represent 10.7% of all boys and 11.5% of all girls

in their sample. The work of Lapouse[13] in the United States is largely in agreement with that of Shepherd.

(3) Looking at cognitive, behavioral and emotional adaptation to the school environment, Kellam and his co-workers[14] studied school children in Chicago. This study defined 13.6% of the children in the sample as severely maladapted, another 19.4% as moderately maladapted and another 36.3% as mildly maladapted. In reviewing the literature, Kellam cited other studies in which proportions of maladaptation range from 10 to 35%.

6. Epidemiological data have been linked to particular social, economic and demographic characteristics which are frequently used to profile populations and which moreover are readily available for any given population.

a) A knowledge of these links will enable a center which does not have available epidemiological data for its own community to make indirect use of existing epidemiological data.

b) To do this, one must know which social, economic and demographic characteristics have been linked to high risk of impairment.

c) Table 4 illustrates the findings relative to age as obtained in the Midtown Manhattan and Stirling County Studies. From these findings, it would appear that the risk of impairment increases with age.

d) From the Midtown Manhattan Study data about the relationship between socioeconomic status and impairment are available (Table 5). Note that those in the lowest socioeconomic strata are most likely to be impaired and those in the highest strata least likely.

e) The Langner Screening Scale study done in New Hampshire has furnished data on the relationships between educational status and impairment and between marital status and impairment (Table 6). Note that in this study educational status and impairment have an inverse relationship. Note that two marital groups, widowed and divorced-separated, have the highest proportions of impaired individuals.

TABLE 4

AGE SPECIFIC RATES IN % FOR IMPAIRMENT
(Midtown Manhattan and Stirling County Studies)

Age	% Impaired Midtown Manhattan	% Impaired Stirling County
20-29	15.3	7.3
30-39	23.2	18.6
40-49	23.2	22.3
50-59	30.8	23.0
60+	N.A.	24.1

TABLE 5

IMPAIRMENT RATES IN % FOR PERSONS IN THE HIGHEST AND LOWEST SOCIOECONOMIC STATUS GROUPS
(Midtown Manhattan Study)

Impairment Category	Highest Socio-economic Status Group	Lowest Socio-economic Status Group
Well	30.0	4.6
Mild and moderate symptom formation	57.5	48.1
Impaired	12.5	47.3

7. In addition to the risk status of various socioeconomic groups, two other related factors bear consideration in the planning process.

   a) Has the particular group been traditionally over-served, underserved or appropriately served relative to its need for services?

   b) Has the particular group been identified as a high priority group for service by funding sources?

TABLE 6

SPECIFIC IMPAIRMENT RATES IN % FOR VARIOUS SUBGROUPS USING THE LANGNER SCALE
New Hampshire (Phillips, 1966)

Specific Category	% Impaired
Education	
Less than High School Graduate	13.6
High School Graduate	7.1
1-3 Years College	2.4
College Graduate	0.0
Marital Status	
Married	7.6
Widowed	12.7
Separated or Divorced	31.6
Never Married	4.8

c) Data for the most commonly considered socioeconomic and demographic variables on these two points are summarized in Table 7, along with a summary of the risk status of each variable.

8. Besides epidemiological data, other related information is of use in the planning process. In determining the necessary size of mental health programs, for instance, the likely number of persons who will seek out services is far more useful than the total number who need services. Such data are available from two sources which will be briefly discussed.

a) In several cities, case registers have been developed. A case register is simply a centralized record-keeping system into which information on every patient seeking services is fed. Registers may be limited to patients admitted only to public programs or may include privately treated patients as well. One such register was developed in Monroe County, New York by Gardner and his associates.[15] Their published data show that yearly admission rates to community mental health services between 1962 and 1967 ranged from 1.2% per year to 1.6%.

b) Another source of such data comes from the so-called prepaid health plans. In such plans, all members pay a yearly fee and are then covered for all or for specified medical and psychiatric needs that may arise through the year. Hence, such plans start with healthy populations and measure how many such persons required and sought out care over a given time period. One of the authors has surveyed the experience of 11 such plans and found yearly utilization rates ranging between 0.6% and 7.2% for outpatient services and between 0.06% and 0.3% for inpatient services.

9. Planning must certainly be a key function of any community mental health center.

   a) In essence, planning is decision-making which is directed in several major directions:

      (1) A determination of what programs should be developed.

      (2) Given the likelihood of limited available resources, a determination of priorities - that is to say, a determination of the priority sequence in which programs are to be assigned resources.

      (3) A determination of where programs should be located. If a series of satellite clinics is to be established, where should each be located and in what sequence should they be established?

      (4) A determination of the specific nature of each program which is established.

      (5) A determination of at which target groups within the population programs should be directed at.

   b) The end product of planning is a plan which details which programs are to be carried out, the sequence in which each will be established, what their nature will be, where each will be located, at whom each will be directed, how much in the way of resources will be devoted to each and finally how each will be evaluated for effectiveness.

TABLE 7

SOCIOECONOMIC AND DEMOGRAPHIC VARIABLES

Social indicator	Is this group at higher than normal risk for mental illness?	Has this group been traditionally overserved or underserved relative to its need for service?	Has this group been identified as a high priority target by funding sources?
Age status: children and adolescents	Available data are sparse but so far do not prove high risk status.	There is much available data to demonstrate that children are frequently underserved.	High priority target group for many funding sources.
Age status: the elderly	Several major studies have shown that impairment increases with age.	There is much available data to demonstrate that the elderly are frequently underserved.	High priority target group for some funding sources.
Ethnic/racial composition: minority group	Available evidence suggests that minorities are at higher than normal risk.	Service to minority groups has been disproportionately high in some areas and disproportionately low in others.	High priority target group for some funding sources.

Economic status: poverty	Available evidence suggests that the poor are at higher than normal risk.	Service to the poor has been disproportionately high in some areas and low in others.	High priority target group for many funding sources.
Social indicator	Is this group at higher than normal risk for mental illness?	Has this group been traditionally overserved or underserved relative to its need for service?	Has this group been identified as a high priority target by funding sources?
Educational status	Available data are very sparse. At least one study shows an inverse relationship.	Some reports suggest that the more educated are more likely to seek out services than are the less educated, creating disparities in service provisions.	Has not been specified as a priority target group by funding sources.
Marital status: separated, divorced or widowed	Studies have shown all three to be high risk groups.	Service to these marital status groups has been very variable.	Has not been specified as priority target group by most funding sources.

c) Planning relies upon three major ingredients:

(1) The capacity to do planning: this comprises a set of skills and expertise that enables the planner to:

(a) Identify and define a set of problems;
(b) Assign priorities to their solutions;
(c) Conceptualize programs to solve them;
(d) Allocate resources between programs on the basis of the priorities which have been set; and
(e) Conceptualize methods to evaluate the programs.

(2) Access to data which enable the planner to identify the problems that are present in the community for which he has the responsibility. Such information is obtained both from census data and from epidemiological data as has already been discussed.

(3) Access to data which assess the effectiveness and efficiency of programs already being carried out. This enables the planner to discard programs that are not working and to replace them with new programs. It enables the planner to selectively assign resources to the most productive programs. These kinds of data will be discussed below in the chapter on evaluation.

d) A hypothetical paradigm for a model community mental health planning process might proceed as follows:

(1) An assessment of community needs either by using a combination of extrapolations from existing epidemiological data and existing census data or by actually carrying out a community survey to directly determine needs.

(2) The establishment, even while the assessment process is still taking place, of services to meet the needs of severely dysfunctional individuals and persons who are in the midst of some crisis situation. This will entail the establishment of a crisis intervention clinic and, linked to it, an inpatient facility.

(3) Having provided for critical needs which cannot await assessments of community need, further planning can take place.

(a) Ambulatory treatment facilities can be established. Their emphasis will depend upon the findings of the needs assessment study.

(b) For instance, communities with large populations of children or elderly patients should certainly consider committing significant proportions of resources to those groups.

(4) Having established an adequate initial base for community treatment, attention might be paid to any residual state hospital population and efforts made to move such patients back to the community where they can be treated in the emerging community care system.

(5) Having begun a system to treat those already impaired, attention could then turn to the establishment of preventive programs. The nature, size and location of these would be determined by the community needs assessment data base.

(6) By this time, the evaluation capacity which has been built into each treatment and preventive program has begun to provide feedback about program effectiveness.

(7) Using such data, decisions can be made regarding:

(a) Unproductive programs which must be modified or abandoned and replaced.

(b) Underserved areas of the community which may require the establishment of satellite clinics or active casefinding or other public education efforts.

(c) Underserved population groups within the community (e.g., a particular minority group) for which special programs may have to be established.

(d) The need to replace existing prevention programs that have done their work or which have not worked with new ones.

10. At this point the first cycle of the planning-implementation-evaluation-plan modification process has taken place. This process will occur over and over again and will insure that, as new evaluation and community needs data flow in, programs will be modified and resources reallocated accordingly.

11. Through all of the above, an active inservice training program has been developed and implemented to insure that the quality and expertise of staff will be constantly upgraded. This must be as integral a part of the planning process as any other part.

12. It remains now to demonstrate how all the data previously presented can actually be used in the planning process.

    a) Epidemiological data can be used to identify high risk population groups.

        (1) As was noted, high levels of impairment have been associated with increasing age, divorced or separated marital status, low educational status and low socioeconomic status. Some of these findings have been replicated in more than one study, others have not. All deserve consideration and further study.

        (2) Once high risk groups have been identified, programs can be devised that direct special attention to them.

        (3) Knowledge about high risk groups that comes from epidemiological data can be used in the process of selecting appropriate "social indicators" for use in assessing mental health needs. In this way, selected items of census data become valuable to the mental health center planning effort as will be discussed.

        (4) Overall estimates of impairment for any catchment area population can be made by applying the rates from the studies cited above to that population. Either overall crude rates or

preferably age-specific rates can be used to calculate the size of the total impaired population. The computation of estimates of the overall size of the impaired population is useful when determining what size delivery system will be necessary to meet total community needs. The best data derived from all the previously mentioned studies seem to indicate that 20 to 25 persons out of every 100 in the population have a significant need for mental health services. Other factors will also determine delivery system size, since the difference between those persons who need services and those who actually seek them out may be considerable.

b) The utilization data which are available from prepaid health plans can be used to project anticipated demand for services and hence be of use in establishing a minimum staffing pattern.
Example: When a mental health center is established, it must estimate its anticipated first year caseload. Using an annual demand rate range of 0.75 - 1.5% obtained from utilization data, a center serving a community of 100,000 persons can make the following calculations:

100,000 persons x 0.75% = 750 persons
100,000 persons x 1.50% = 1500 persons

Anticipated range of persons seeking service in the first year of operation is likely to be between 750 and 1500.

c) Census data can be used to weigh the importance of various population characteristics in program development and implementation. By asking whether children or old persons or poor persons represent sizable proportions of a community's population, the appropriateness of developing special programs to serve such groups can be determined.
Example: Easy geographic access to clinic facilities and a readily adjustable fee schedule are important considerations for any center serving significant proportions of poor persons. Census data can determine the proportion of poor persons living in an area.
Example: The need for bilingual staff must be gauged by the presence or absence of a significant

number of persons whose primary language is not English. The numbers of such persons can be determined from census data.

d) Census data can also be used to establish denominators for various subgroups within the population. The need for such data will become more apparent later in the chapter on evaluation when utilization rates of different population subgroups must be calculated.

e) Census data can be mapped in order to produce a visual display of a population distribution for any particular demographic, social or economic characteristic. This provides a particularly vivid means of revealing where high concentrations of a particular characteristic and hence high risk groups are to be found within the catchment area. Such map displays can be used effectively to plan and to implement mental health programs in a number of ways:

(1) Decisions related to site selection for primary centers or for satellite clinics can utilize these kinds of data.

(a) Site selection can be based on the location of areas of greatest population density which can be demonstrated by mapping.

(b) Site selection can be based on the whereabouts of particular high priority target populations. High concentration of such populations can be demonstrated using the mapping procedure.

(2) Decisions concerning where to mount public information and education programs, consultation programs, casefinding efforts and prevention programs can utilize census data maps in similar fashion.

f) To summarize, then, epidemiological, utilization and census data can all be used to determine the whos, whats and wheres of service requirements.

REFERENCES

1. Srole, L., Langner, T., Michael, S., Opler, M., Rennie, T. Mental Health in the Metropolis - The Midtown Manhattan Study. New York: McGraw-Hill, 1962.

2. Leighton, D., Harding, J., Macklin, D., MacMillan, A., and Leighton, A. The Character of Danger - The Stirling County Study. Volume III. New York: Basic Books, 1963.

3. Langner, T. A Twenty-Two Item Screening Score of Psychiatry Symptoms Indicating Impairment. J. Hlth. and Human Behav. 3:269-276, 1962.

4. Manis, J., Brawer, M., Hunt, C. and Kercher, L. Estimating the Prevalence of Mental Illness. Am. Sociolog. Rev. 29:84-89, 1964.

5. Phillips, D. The "True Prevalence" of Mental Illness in a New England State. Comm. Mental Hlth. J. 2:35-40, 1966.

6. Meile, R. The Twenty-Two Index of Psychophysiological Disorder: Psychological or Organic Symptoms? Soc. Science and Med. 6:125-135, 1972.

7. Gaitz, C. and Scott, J. Age and the Measurement of Mental Health. J. Hlth. and Soc. Behav. 13:55-67, 1973.

8. Pasamanik, B. A Survey of Mental Disease in an Urban Population: An Approach to Total Prevalence Rates. Arch. Gen. Psychiatr. 5:151-155, 1961.

9. Cole, M., Branch, C. and Orla, M. Mental Illness. A Survey of Community Rates. Arch. Neurol. and Psychiatr. 77:393-398, 1957.

10. Tischler, G., Henisz, T., Myers, J. and Boswell, P. Utilization of Mental Health Services - Patienthood and the Prevalence of Symptomology in the Community. Arch. Gen. Psychiatr. 32:411-416, 1975.

11. Langner, T., Gersten, J., McCarthy, E. and Eisenberg, J. A Screening Inventory for Assessing Psychiatric Impairment in Children 6 to 18. J. Consult. and Clin. Psychol. 44:286-296, 1976.

12. Shepherd, M., Oppenheim, B. and Mitchell, S. Childhood Behavior and Mental Health. New York: Grune and Stratton, 1971.

13. Lapouse, R. and Monk, M. An Epidemiologic Study of Behavior Characteristics in Children. Am. J. Public Hlth. 48:1134-1144, 1958.

14. Kellan, S., Branch, J., Agrawal, K. and Ensminger, M. Mental Health and Going to School. Chicago: University of Chicago Press, 1975.

15. Gardner, E. The Use of a Psychiatric Case Register in the Planning and Evaluation of a Mental Health Program. Psychiatric Epidemiology and Mental Health Planning. R. Monroe, et al. (Eds.). Washington, D.C.: American Psychiatric Association, 1967, pp. 259-281.

CHAPTER 4

CLINICAL TREATMENT APPROACHES IN COMMUNITY MENTAL HEALTH

Donald G. Langsley, M.D.

1. Introduction

a) This chapter is meant to outline the practical operations of clinical treatment in a community mental health center (CMHC). It assumes that the center has a responsibility to a population (catchment area), that it offers a variety of treatment services, and that it is operated by a multi-disciplinary mental health team.

b) There are basic assessment approaches to the intake process. We assume that patient symptoms, malfunctions and "problems" are not simply associated with the diagnosis of the identified patient. It is important to know the reasons why a patient seeks help (or is brought in for help), the problems or symptoms that initiated the request for help, and how a given setting may effectively evaluate the problem as well as potential treatment-management. It is also important to understand the family and/or other social support systems in the patient's environment.

c) Treatment is often nonspecific and directed toward problems or social systems, rather than being a specific approach associated with a given diagnosis which one sometimes finds in physical medicine.

d) Treatment may be planned and offered by an individual or a mental health team. When offered by a multi-disciplinary team, it must be recognized that various members of that team have generalized (overlapping) as well as specialized skills. These must be taken into account in the planning and implementation of treatment.

e) Treatment-management varies in different settings. The ideal CMHC has a variety of settings, offering treatment designed to meet the needs of a given patient. These include (at least) crisis-emergency services, outpatient services, partial hospitalization and inpatient services. Treatment plans will often be carried out in phases - one might imagine that, for a given patient, one aspect of the treatment would be carried on in <u>each</u> of the above settings.

f) Certain clinical conditions require specialized approaches to psychotherapy and/or pharmacotherapy or other somatic treatment. This chapter will offer treatment suggestions for a variety of the more common conditions.

2. <u>What to treat: the intake process</u>

a) <u>Initial contact.</u> The initial contact may be made by telephone, by the patient walking into an emergency service or crisis center, or by the patient being brought in by family members, friends or police. The patient may be referred by another physician, by a social service agency or by a minister. Whatever the source or route, the initial contact is often the most important opportunity to be of help. An expressed willingness to help, the immediate availability of help, and the manner in which the initial contact is made will influence the total treatment process.

(1) These points of initial contact are often conducted in busy and stressful settings. It is

important for the person answering the phone or making the contact to explain to an individual requesting help that it may take a few minutes, but that someone will be available shortly. Phone calls may have to be returned. Triage decisions may have to be made about which situations are the most critical. But this must be done in a manner which indicates that the emergency service staff member is attentive and will be of whatever help possible.

(2) When the initial contact is with a clerk trained to get demographic information and/or financial evaluations, it is especially important to teach that clerk to be sensitive to the immediate needs of the patient. The mental health professional who will see the patient should be consulted if there is any question.

b) The setting. This initial contact may take place in any of the settings previously mentioned. Telephone "hot line" settings were first developed to prevent suicide, but have come to offer around-the-clock help for a variety of problems. Often they are used by lonely people wanting someone to talk with them. But sometimes, they are used by persons truly in crisis. The emergency psychiatric service located in the general hospital emergency room is a natural location for a "hot line" service. In addition to being a resource long viewed as the place to go for health emergencies, the presence of mental health personnel in that setting makes it possible for them to consult with physicians and nurses dealing with what may only appear to be a physical problem. It is also advantageous to use this setting because the patient comes to a general hospital emergency room for any type of health problem and, presumably, this association reduces the stigma of mental disorder.

(1) Nonhospital crisis service in a CMHC. Some community mental health centers which are not hospital-based offer their crisis services in nonhospital settings. Here the staff may rotate availability for serving "drop-in" patients requiring immediate attention. In cities where there are many mental health centers,

an alternative arrangement allows availability of crisis intervention during normal business hours at each of the centers. Because of the staffing requirements and expense of 24-hour services, there is frequently a single central night and weekend emergency service - often in the emergency room of a public hospital. Since the peak of activity in such centers is generally from 4:00 p. m. to midnight, the central emergency service may see a large proportion of the cases seeking help.

(2) Social service agencies are another type of setting which offers immediate aid or "walk-in" services. Welfare agencies and courts see a large number of individuals who require such help.

c) Referral pathway is a matter which the psychiatrist or other mental health professional should consider. Understanding the channels through which the patient came to the emergency service and identifying those who made the referral will often throw light on the immediate problem. This information should be sought early in the contact. Along with the first question ("How can I help you?" or "What is the problem?"), additional queries such as: "How did you happen to come here?" and "Why did you come at this particular time?" are key questions for the initial contact. The answers to these questions will often help to identify the immediate problem, who thought it to be a problem and what motivation the patient has for seeking help with whatever he defines the problem to be.

d) Definition of the problem. The presenting problem may be far more complicated than a symptom. It may be an acute illness. It may be a life crisis of some sort confronting a person who has been previously labeled a "mental patient", or in one never so labeled. It may be a reality problem ("Where can I find housing?" or "... a job?"). It may represent some type of decompensation in a person with a chronic mental disorder (the chronic schizophrenic who goes off medication and becomes delusional again). It may be an acute or recently developing mental disorder, as with depressive illness or an anxiety attack. Whatever it is, the first efforts of the initial interviewer will be to hear and to understand the present problem. Psychiatrists and other mental health professionals are too often concerned with the past - with developmental events from childhood or with patterns of interpersonal difficulties. But at this point, effort and attention should be concerned with the present-immediate problem. Later, the problem can be put in the context of the patient's life and personality style. Questions and speculations can then be made about the cause of the problem. The problem's definition should focus on the immediate symptoms and/or complaints and on the functional disabilities associated with that problem.

(1) Symptoms or complaints. They will be elicited by asking what the problem is - or how the person needs help. The interviewer must then listen for awhile to permit the patient to tell his own story. This chapter will not try to cover all the techniques of interviewing and evaluating (for that information, a textbook of clinical psychiatry is more appropriate). But it is useful to remind the interviewer that active and empathic listening is required at this point. Attention must be paid exclusively to the patient, without interruption by the interviewer. An occasional question asking for clarification, or a summary comment to indicate briefly that what is being communicated is being heard or understood, will help. But this is not the time to ask closed-ended questions, or to interrupt the flow of the patient's communication. After listening for awhile, the interviewer may begin to ask questions to obtain further details about the present problem, but these, too, should be open-ended. As the interview progresses, the questions requiring more "yes" or "no" responses may be helpful, but not in the beginning.

(2) Functional disabilities. The symptoms or problems may reflect a change in the patient's usual functioning. The important information to seek is about change. If the patient had been working regularly or had been able to

carry on a variety of social relationships and this suddenly changed, that is different from the patient who had not worked for years and had been a social recluse. One should look for information about change in functional adaptation in areas of: (a) work or school or homemaking responsibilities; (b) social contacts with family, friends, clubs or organizations; and/or (c) relationships with key family members or friends; as well as for the presence or absence of symptoms of mental disorder.

(3) Specific problem areas should be of concern to the interviewer. These include:

(a) The potential for suicide or self-harm of a more subtle nature. Information about suicide thoughts as well as the presence or absence of a suicidal intent or plans are obviously important. But some people harm themselves in a more hidden fashion, e.g., repeated accidents. The most serious suicide risk is the older male who is living alone, has a drinking problem, may have a debilitating physical illness, and lacks hope for the future. Younger women are more likely to make a suicide attempt, but their efforts are frequently not as lethal as those of the first-described individual. Suicide is increasing among adolescents and even among pre-adolescent children. It is always important to consider the patient's potential for suicide. Identifying such potential may be lifesaving. Though one does not ask it as the first question, almost any person considering suicide will reveal that intent if skillfully interviewed. Most interviewers go through a series of questions including queries as to whether the patient feels depressed or "down"; whether the patient feels that life is so difficult that it is not worth living; whether the patient has considered harming or killing himself - and if so, whether he has a specific plan; whether he has a means (guns, pills, etc.); and whether there have been prior suicide attempts by the patient or members of the family.

(b) Impaired impulse control. More and more frequently the patient with problems of actual or potential violent behavior is brought to the psychiatry emergency service. This situation calls for keen judgment, since the responsibility for preventing harm to others is seen (by some) as even more important than preventing injury by the patient to himself. Our society is more frequently made aware of violence toward children, violence toward spouses, etc., and there are legal requirements for reporting abuse to children. Specialized community facilities have been developed for sheltering abused spouses or children. In judging the potential for violence, one must consider any underlying illness. A psychosis makes some persons more violence-prone since there is a lack of ego control over such impulses. Alcohol complicates the management of many types of violence. The use of alcohol removes controls and inhibitions in quarrelling family members and couples. In evaluating the possibilities of violent behavior, the interviewer should seek data about prior violent episodes. This includes a history of childhood episodes of fire-setting and/or cruelty to animals. Other essential data should include inquiries about the availability of a gun, use of drugs other than alcohol, and the usual frustration tolerance of the patient. Schizoid persons who are suspicious and paranoid are of special concern since they may lash out impulsively. The offer of help and/or a "show of force" will often lend controls to the patient, and they are generally accepted.

(c) Inability to care for basic needs. The interviewer should determine whether the patient has recently been able to care for his own personal physical needs such as food, shelter, clothing, etc. Patients with acute or chronic brain syndromes may be in danger of losing their lives through the loss of these key abilities.

(d) Social dysfunctioning. Although any change in social behavior was mentioned above as an important area of consideration, it is useful to highlight topics which should be covered in questioning: Is the patient one who had previously been involved with others, but who has suddenly become a hermit? Have friends and relatives become inaccessible through external circumstances? Has the patient begun to associate with individuals who are likely to be harmful to him? Individuals may be brought to the mental health center (usually adolescent or aged people) because of the family's concern over new friends or associates who are thought to be harmful.

e) Precipitating stresses. The concept of a crisis or sudden change in ability to function is associated with susceptibility and recent stress. The patient should be queried about recent changes or stresses in his life. Acute psychiatric illness may follow such life stresses as change in family composition (through death, divorce or additions), illness of a close friend or family member, loss of job, financial distress, and many others. Associations between stress and the development of acute physical and mental illness have been shown in the work of several investigators, including Rahe and Holmes and the Dohrenwends.

(1) Why now? is a question which may broaden understanding of the current problem. The interviewer should try to understand why the patient seeks help at this particular time. Conditions which are long-standing may be the subject of complaint, but it may be a recent marital complication, job loss, interpersonal crisis or similar event which is the

reason for seeking help at this time. A classic example is the person of long-standing homosexual orientation who arrives at the treatment center saying that he has a sexual orientation problem - when in fact the reason for seeking treatment now is the breakup of a relationship and not the homosexuality itself.

3. Who is to be treated? Though there is usually an "identified patient", the interviewer should scan the immediate social field of that patient and look carefully at the person(s) who brought the patient to the emergency service or clinic intake. This requires a systems frame of reference and attention to the patient's social interactions, as well as to biopsychological conditions.

   a) The patient. The identified patient should be evaluated in his own right. This includes attention to physical as well as psychological and social problems. The person who complains of fatigue, loss of energy, sleep disturbance and similar vague events may have a physical illness. But these are also symptoms of depression. It is of value to have the initial evaluation done either by a psychiatrist or by a combination of a nonpsychiatric physician and a mental health professional.

   b) Family, spouse, significant others should also be the focus of attention. The "important others" in a patient's life are important both for the role that they may have played in precipitating the reaction in the patient and for the help and social support they can offer the patient. They may give information which the patient will not reveal. When the patient is obtunded or otherwise unable to give information, it is vital to see another person. The other sources may confirm, extend or alter the data available for determining what the current problem is. The presence of a social support system will also help determine what course of treatment the mental health professional will take. The depressed patient with suicidal thoughts who lives alone without support will more likely require hospitalization than the same patient who has a family, roommate or friends who will stay with him.

c) Caretakers. Patients may be brought to the intake process by caretakers such as the staff of a residential center, a teacher, a minister or a staff member from a social service agency. These caretakers should be interviewed for information and help in determining resources available for disposition. In addition, the caretaker may also require help. The caretaker who has watched a crisis or illness develop and who finally reaches a point of asking for outside help may be feeling guilty or upset about his inability to master the situation. The same caretaker may require counseling about managing the patient in the future. By enlisting the aid of the caretaker at this point, and by indicating optimism about the patient's chances of recovery, the disposition and future course of the patient may be improved.

4. Where to treat? Assessment and treatment may take place in a variety of settings in the CMHC. The location and process of the assessment and treatment planning have been previously outlined. Once the treatment plan has been developed, it may take place in one of the following settings:

a) Telephone crisis treatment is one possible avenue for crisis intervention, especially as it applies to acute and short-term problems. It is easier for someone to get help on the phone if they have had prior contact with the helping agency. An individual in therapy with a staff member of the CMHC may seek telephone aid when a crisis arises at night or on the weekend. Similarly, an individual with prior experience as a patient in that agency may be helped through an immediate problem. Questions about medication may be resolved on the telephone. Issues about referrals or information about other treatment programs may be given. It is more difficult for the person who has not had prior contact with the emergency service to be helped by simple phone contact - especially if the crisis is a serious one. If the person is known to the system but not to the staff member on the phone, it is still advisable to persuade the patient to come in for a face-to-face interview.

b) Home or residential care settings are other possible locations for treatment. They are used when the CMHC has a traveling team or a staff member who can make "house calls". Mobile crisis intervention or brief treatment in the home or residential care setting is thereby possible. When patients are bedridden or when there is some reason why the patient cannot travel to the center or emergency service, it may be possible to avert an admission to the hospital if a staff member can go to the patient and consult with other members of the family (if the patient lives at home) or with caretakers (if the patient lives in an organized residential center).

c) Jails or other correctional institutions. Treatment may have to be carried on in a jail or juvenile detention center when inmates of such institutions require mental care. In such settings there is usually a consultant (or team) who visits the institution regularly, does evaluations and makes recommendations about the management of serious problems within the institution. Because of security considerations, the institution is generally reluctant to transfer an inmate to a mental hospital. Instead, officials may agree to allow treatment of inmates in the prison setting.

d) Emergency psychiatric service or crisis intervention unit. Many of the procedures described in Sections 2 and 3 can be carried on in the emergency service or crisis intervention unit, where patients may be scheduled for return visits. These units too often consider themselves evaluation-disposition units and should take on the additional responsibility of providing brief outpatient crisis intervention for individuals or families. It has been demonstrated that outpatient family crisis treatment averaging 5 or 6 visits (plus phone calls) can act as an effective alternative to mental hospital admission. Crisis intervention for individuals or families can be of great value as the definitive treatment in managing a crisis and its resolution. In addition to this type of outpatient crisis intervention, some emergency psychiatry units make use of "holding beds". This approach utilizes the emergency room for up to 24 or 36 hours of acute treatment in the emergency room. It often averts an otherwise unnecessary hospital admission. For the patient who has made a suicide gesture and is recovering from medical treatment for an overdose, and for other types of acute crisis in which observation and support for several hours are necessary, this type of approach has been found to be extremely helpful.

e) Outpatient clinics are another setting for treatment. Actually they are the classic settings for individuals with less urgent psychological problems. The more profoundly ill patients who may require hospitalization are referred to outpatient treatment after the hospital phase. Outpatient clinics are generally one of the more important parts of the CMHC and account for a large proportion of the clinical activities of the center. They offer a variety of treatment programs - mostly psychotherapeutic or a combination of psychotherapy and medication. They offer short- and long-term treatment. The ideal outpatient clinic would be able to offer brief therapy and intensive, long-term psychotherapy, including psychoanalysis. They should be able to treat adults, children, married couples and families. They should have specialized programs such as are needed for alcoholics, chronic schizophrenics needing aftercare, adolescents and the aged. They should have close connections with the emergency service intake process and the inpatient service, or have a partial hospitalization program. The outpatient clinic is almost invariably staffed by a multi-disciplinary team. In addition to direct treatment services, they may also offer mental health consultation and education services, but those programs are discussed elsewhere in this volume.

f) Partial hospitalization is a term which may include day-long hospitalization, night-long hospitalization, or any other variation on the theme of less-than-24-hour inpatient services. Usually, it takes the form of day hospitalization between the hours of 8:00 a.m. and 5:00 p.m., Monday through Friday. Individuals who can live at home in a family style setting frequently receive this type of treatment. The treatment program generally includes individual and group psychotherapy, medication, milieu, activities therapy, and all other treatments generally available in a 24-hour hospital. It has been shown by the Fort Logan group, the Albert Einstein group and many others, that most patients who would otherwise require 24-hour hospitalization can be treated in this type of setting. The partial hospitalization approach may be either an alternative to 24-hour hospitalization in order to avoid such admission, or a transition measure for those who have been hospitalized in a traditional setting and who require this intermediate step before being discharged. Such programs are more typically found in urban than in rural areas because of the traveling required. The family must be able and willing to cooperate with partial hospitalization for it to be effective. The patient cannot have a condition requiring segregation from addictive substances (drugs, alcohol), nor can the patient be so disoriented that he cannot function on a part-time basis in the community setting. Schizophrenics, in particular, can benefit from partial hospitalization. Day hospitals provide socialization and can enhance self-esteem. This approach also permits the patient to remain in the family for a part of the time, and thus continues an important social support system. The cost of such hospitalization is considerably less than the cost of 24-hour treatment; but to date, third party carriers and government programs have been reluctant to embrace the concept and cover the cost in their health care programs. Their concern is that the day hospital is a new service for individuals who would not otherwise require hospitalization.

g) The inpatient service - the psychiatric hospital. The 24-hour mental hospital can be a specialized ward of a general hospital, a private psychiatric hospital, or a state mental hospital (including VA hospitals). Any or all the above may relate to a CMHC and may serve as the inpatient service for the center (although VA hospitals are limited to serving veterans, exclusively). Hospitals are the preferred setting for treating the more seriously ill, as they provide a better means of protecting the patient, the family and society from potential dangers. Hospitalization of a patient may be required if:

(1) The patient is suicidal or potentially dangerous to others;

(2) The patient cannot attend to his basic needs (such as food, shelter, clothing, etc.);

(3) There are no external social supports which would permit treatment outside the hospital;

(4) Hospitalization is needed to initiate a therapeutic relationship which may be continued on an outpatient basis; and/or

(5) The family is exhausted with the problems of managing this particular patient, or the patient needs to be removed from the family because they are particularly pathogenic.

There are disadvantages to hospitalization, including: (a) the stigma often associated with the label "mental patient" (a person is not a "mental patient" until he has been a patient in a mental hospital); (b) the tendency of hospitals to permit or encourage regression and hospitalization; and (c) the difficulties faced by the family when a patient is removed from the home and admitted to a hospital, especially one located some distance from the home. Some hospitals have programs designed to perform immediate evaluation and short-term treatment, with goals of reconstituting the patient, alleviating acute symptoms and returning the patient to his prior level of functioning. Other hospitals have more ambitious goals: instead of settling for symptomatic improvement, they aim for rehabilitation of long-term problems and endeavor to help the patient achieve levels of skill and functioning which represent his potential. These rehabilitative goals come closer to the concept of "cure", yet we are often reminded that more conclusive evidence is needed to prove that "cure" actually takes place. One of the problems of the inpatient program in the CMHC is that the center may have to use an inpatient service located some distance from the rest of the program. Because hospitals are considerably more expensive than outpatient services, various centers often collaborate with each other in using a common inpatient service (often on a contractual basis). To achieve continuity of care, staff from the center must travel to their hospitalized patients. Hospitals, on the other hand, are geared toward working with a full-time staff, and their organization requires at least a "core" of such persons - psychiatrists, social workers, nurses, psychologists. If the hospital is a long-term care institution (such as a distant state mental hospital for the chronic schizophrenic), the center soon realizes that it has to settle for substantially less patient contact, exclusion from the processes of treatment planning and implementation and, eventually, dependence upon written or telephoned reports of the patient's progress. In such situations, the center staff do not control the length of stay and, at best, can only try to participate in the discharge planning before a patient is actually released.

h) Other settings - the chronic patient. A major disappointment in the community mental health movement has been the result of chronic patient deinstitutionalization before the community has developed the specialized programs necessary for receiving and treating the former hospital patient. For the chronic patient to be managed successfully in the community (by which is meant, that the chronic patient is not simply ignored or placed in board-and-care settings where he may be neglected), there must be a panoply of specialized services functioning in the community and able to accommodate the deinstitutionalized patient. Significant among those services are the subacute hospitals, or 24-hour residential treatment settings where the proper care can be provided for several months. Other specialized programs of rehabilitation-resocialization which a community should provide for the chronic patient are crisis intervention services, medication-aftercare clinics, a range of supervised living settings, and a method for tracking patients who might otherwise "fall between the cracks". Aggressive and continuous follow-up is a necessary component of chronic patient treatment.

5. What kind of treatment?

a) Psychotherapy. Psychotherapy is the mainstay therapy of most mental health professionals. However, its nature is so complex that efforts to define it; to explain specifically how to do it, for what condition, for which patient; and to demonstrate the efficacy and safety of this form of treatment will inevitably meet with some frustrations. There are 120-140 different schools or approaches to psychotherapy. An often-quoted definition of psychotherapy is: "the informed and planful application of techniques derived from established psychological principles, by persons qualified through training and experience to understand these principles and to apply these techniques, with the intention of assisting individuals to modify such personal characteristics as feelings, values, attitudes and behaviors which are judged by the therapist to be maladaptive or maladjustive." There are individual psychotherapies, family or marital psychotherapies, and group psychotherapies. Each may have the goal of support or reconstruction/re-education. The most carefully defined psychotherapy is psychoanalysis, where the "classic" model is highly explicated and agreed upon. Though there have been complaints about prospective and retrospective research on its effects and usefulness, the fact is that there is a broad literature outlining the types of patients and problems for which psychoanalysis is useful and can be expected to produce certain outcomes. A recent review of the research on outcome in psychotherapy (in which Glass, et al. collected and analyzed some 500 published reports on the controlled study of psychotherapy) suggests that psychotherapy - regardless of brand - always has some positive effect. The average patient who received therapy was shown to have been better off (after treatment) than 75% of those who did not receive treatment. Patients who received psychotherapy for fear and anxiety showed more improvement than 83% of the untreated controls. Psychotherapy alone is generally not used for schizophrenia, affective psychoses, alcoholism or similar conditions, and it has been questioned in the treatment of severe obsessive-compulsive disorders. It is, however, more useful for anxiety states, fears and phobias and less serious depression. A recent study suggests that with cognitive psychotherapy, patients also do better with therapy alone than with only drugs.

Psychotherapy depends on an alliance between patient and therapist. However, this alliance alone is not psychotherapy; it is only a requisite component of such therapy. Skilled psychotherapy requires a knowledge of the psychological situation in which the patient finds himself, a plan under which the psychological situation may be altered, and a knowledge of techniques to be applied. It must be a planned rather than an intuitive or "seat of the pants" operation. Good intentions and a sympathetic or empathic attitude on the therapist's part are not enough, although these contributions are essential. Before one can reach an appropriate level of skill in psychotherapy, years of study and supervised practice must come first. The fact that it seems so simple and natural (after all, psychotherapy consists of talking and listening, and most people can do both) gives some the impression that anyone can perform psychotherapy. Because of this misconception, and because there are no impressive technical machines or special operating rooms associated with it, too many unskilled individuals attempt to "practice" psychotherapy. Theoretical disagreements among psychotherapists have led to the development of the 120-140 "schools" of psychotherapy, but most of those approaches are based on an individual's belief system rather than empirical data or scientific evidence. Psychotherapy is a special skill to be learned and applied in the same manner as other scientific treatment, and the supposition that anyone in a CMHC can do any variety of psychotherapy is dangerously false. The humanitarian impulse to offer therapy when one encounters a person with severe psychological illness must be exercised with the same precautions and the same judgment one would use in rendering aid to the victim of a serious auto accident. In both instances, there is a high possibility of unseen, internal injuries which can be made worse by well-intentioned but inappropriate assistance. What may sometimes qualify as "psychologically therapeutic" (a friendly ear, a comforting bartender) is <u>not</u> psychotherapy.

This manual is not intended to be a mini-textbook of psychotherapy. The reader who wants to learn more about it should consult the many textbooks and multi-volume encyclopedias devoted to this topic. The reader who wants to practice it should be reminded that responsible, effective skill in psychotherapy comes only with supervised experience.

Psychotherapy is not meant to be limited to the one-to-one (therapist-to-patient) relationship. It is also helpful to assign individual patients to groups, or to treat families or married couples together.

(1) Group psychotherapy may have as its goals the support and education of its members or the exploration of their repressed or unconscious conflicts. (Group therapy may also be combined with individual therapy.) A variety of approaches may be applied in group therapy, including psychodrama, transactional analysis and gestalt therapy, as well as psychoanalytically-oriented treatment.

(a) Guidance groups are used for the purpose of teaching and inspiring changes in behavior (e.g., alcoholics or parents of retarded children).

(b) Counseling groups are used for the purpose of ego-support and will often focus on the effects of conscious and unconscious attitudes in interpersonal relations. (Many once-a-week groups operate in this manner.)

(c) Expressive or analytically-oriented groups focus on unconscious forces. These forces are drawn out through an inactive leader who uses the development of transferences within the group to help insight develop.

(d) Marathon groups use long sessions (3-12 hours) or a total weekend to open communication and develop group cohesiveness.

For all types of group therapy, a homogeneous arrangement is usually preferred - homogeneous in terms of age and/or pathology. Groups are less useful for those with acute situational problems or for individuals who are so acutely ill that they can neither trust sufficiently to deal with an outpatient group nor manage the social interaction required.

(2) Family or marital therapy uses the natural support system of the family and explores some of the problems which may have precipitated psychiatric illness in the "identified

patient". It is designed to help the whole family, not just the patient. One technique seeks to enhance mutual support through facilitation of communication. Sometimes, however, it is necessary to alter disturbed roles and inter-family coalitions (e.g., structural family therapy as described by Minuchin); and in such cases, the therapist also functions as role model and educator. There are a variety of approaches in this field (as in group and individual psychotherapy) and some therapists focus on reconstruction of important past events while others concentrate on the present. Family therapy is indicated when the problem seems to be a system difficulty disturbing the family unit. Conflict and dissatisfaction between a husband and wife respond well to conjoint treatment. When a child or adolescent is the identified patient, involvement of the whole family is especially useful. Family therapy is more complicated and even contra-indicated when there is impending dissolution of the family, or when the identified patient is attempting to emancipate himself from the family.

(3) Individual psychotherapy is the approach most frequently used. It may be conducted on a short-term (crisis-oriented) basis, as in focal psychotherapy; or it may need to be long-term psychotherapy or even psychoanalysis. As noted above, there are many schools and many approaches to psychotherapy, each requiring careful evaluation and skill in treatment. Individual psychotherapy can also be behavioral in its orientation. Behavior therapy assumes that psychopathology is the result of learned, involuntarily acquired, undesirable "habits". The goals are to replace such ineffective habits with more adaptive behaviors.

   (a) Desensitization is one approach found useful in phobic conditions.

   (b) Implosive therapy and flooding have been used for treating anxiety. (The patient is exposed to anxiety-provoking situations for long periods of time.)

(c) Assertive training is designed to resolve interpersonal problems and improve social interaction.

(d) Operant approaches, including reinforcement and aversive conditioning, have been used to inhibit maladaptive behavior and reinforce the desired adaptive behavior.

(e) Biofeedback has been used to alter autonomic responses with the help of physiological feedback. It has been used with hypertension, migraine and similar conditions.

(f) Cognitive behavior therapy is an approach that attempts to terminate or change negative thinking. It has been used to help depressed patients change recurrent negative thought patterns, to emphasize the positive and to try to increase self-esteem.

b) Milieu therapy is conducted in a hospital or partial-hospital setting. It has been used with all types of hospitalized patients, but the milieu (or therapeutic community) method has been particularly emphasized for those with personality disorders and those with chronic schizophrenia. Milieu therapy differs from other approaches in that both the group within the institution and the total institutional/social environment are used to influence the patient's personal autonomy and to change behavior. Some milieu approaches derive from studies of institutions and their effects on long-term patients. It was found that a syndrome of hospitalism develops from the experience of mental hospitalization. Staff conflicts have serious consequences for the behavior of patients, and patients themselves influence the behavior and responses of staff. Systems theory and group process have enhanced understanding of psychiatric wards and have contributed to the improvement of milieu therapy. The hospital should no longer be seen as a series of spaces for containing patients while medication or other "treatment" is administered. Hospital staff cannot simply view the patient as a passive object to which some type of therapy is administered; rather, the patient is to be viewed as one who participates in the process of helping his own adaptation, and one who takes some responsibility for helping other patients (and staff). All events on the ward are regarded as potential opportunities for furthering the planned therapeutic effort. Community meetings are used to demonstrate that patients can participate in decisions which affect them. Open expression of feelings encourages communication, while specific effort is directed toward helping each patient improve his self-esteem. Milieu therapy is not used by itself, but in combination with psychotherapy (individual, group or family) and with somatic therapy (medication, ECT). Schizophrenics have been shown to benefit from pharmacotherapy, individual psychotherapy and the social therapies available in the milieu.

c) <u>Somatic therapies (other than pharmacotherapy).</u> Insulin coma therapy or subcoma therapy was used for many years for schizophrenia. Psychoactive drugs have largely superseded this approach, however, and it is rarely seen today. The convulsive therapies began with the use of camphor and metrazol to induce seizures. These were replaced by electroconvulsive therapy (ECT) which continues to be effective in the treatment of serious depression and (less frequently) schizophrenia. Flurothyl was later found to induce seizures as effectively as ECT, but was more difficult to use. Today, modified ECT - combining atropine, short-acting anesthetics and muscle relaxants (succinylcholine) along with inhalation of oxygen to reduce hypoxia - is a routine procedure. Despite recent legal and political attacks, ECT remains a useful treatment for psychotic depressions - especially when antidepressants have been tried without success - and it is of particular value in the treatment of acutely suicidal patients. ECT has also been effective in alleviating acute mania. Some clinicians have been enthusiastic about ECT for schizophrenics, especially those with catatonic excitement or who have failed to respond to a variety of antipsychotic medications. There are practically no proven, absolute contraindications, and ECT's side effects can be easily controlled. Most clinicians have found that the amnesia associated with ECT does not persist, and that memory generally returns after 4-8 weeks. The technique of using unilateral electrodes over the nondominant hemisphere has significantly reduced ECT-associated amnesia. This procedure should be administered in a hospital.

6. Pharmacotherapy. This section will be concerned only with antipsychotic drugs (neuroleptics), antidepressants, lithium and anti-anxiety medications.

   a) These are all potent agents and must be prescribed by one who is familiar with their use and legally authorized to prescribe drugs. Nonphysician mental health professionals should have a reasonable knowledge of the classes of compounds in these drugs, how they are used and what their potential side effects can be. However, the practice of having non-MD's decide upon their use and prepare the prescription for a physician to sign is not only potentially illegal, but also dangerous to patients. The physician who signs such prescriptions without periodically examining the patient face-to-face and without giving careful attention to all aspects of the patient's physical and mental health is not practicing an acceptable quality of medicine.

   b) These medications have varying effects on different patients. There are average, but no standard doses; each patient's medication must be individualized. Side effects must be carefully observed, and any medications prescribed for altering those side effects must also be individually balanced because they are likewise quite potent.

   c) Dual compounds are less easily regulated than single compounds; therefore, single compounds are preferred.

   d) Drug interactions are a frequent problem, and all other medications being taken by a patient should be known to the physician. Some drugs potentiate one another and some can be extremely dangerous when combined with others. Drug interaction complications include:

      (1) Alteration of absorption;
      (2) Changes in drug metabolism and/or excretion rates;

(3) Receptor site synergism or antagonism; and/or
(4) Toxicity which manifests itself in cardiac, metabolic, neurologic, psychiatric, renal, hepatic and other systemic complications

e) The success of pharmacotherapy depends not only on the drug, but also on the relationship between the physician and patient. Placebo effects influence drug effect. The cooperation of the patient (sometimes called "compliance") is essential. Patients often adjust doses, omit one or several doses, or simply discontinue the drug because of side effects, denial of their illness, or problems in their relationship with the physician. The practice of giving patients written instructions for taking medications and of obtaining from them an informed consent document can be very helpful - sometimes even essential in obtaining the patient's cooperation.

f) Antipsychotic drugs. These are used for schizophrenia or other psychoses. Occasionally, they are used as anti-emetics, and to potentiate analgesics.

(1) They are classified as:

(a) Phenothiazines (e.g., chlorpromazine, trifluoperazine, thioridazine or fluphenazine);
(b) Butyrophenones (e.g., haloperidol);
(c) Thioxanthenes (e.g., chlorprothixene); and
(d) Dibenzoxazepines (e.g., loxapine)

(2) The procedure used is to give the drug in divided oral doses 2-4x daily with gradual increases every 3-4 days until a therapeutic response or intolerable side effects are reached. Doses are always individualized. After 2-3 weeks, they can be given in a single daily dose at night. Maintenance dosages are individually determined according to clinical conditions, but drug holidays may be useful in avoiding long-term or permanent neurologic side effects such as tardive dyskinesia.

(a) Drugs may be given intramuscularly in acute cases at 1-6 hour intervals, after which the patient should be switched to oral doses. Perphenazine or haloperidol is preferred for IM use. The depot medications (fluphenazine decanoate) are useful for noncompliant patients needing maintenance therapy and may be useful in patients who absorb drugs poorly following oral administration.

(b) Standard psychiatry or pharmacology textbooks should be consulted for details on doses, side effects, contraindications, etc.

(3) Side effects of the antipsychotics include:

(a) Extrapyramidal reactions (dystonias, rigidity, tremor, akinesias, akasthisia). They may be modified with antiparkinson drugs (anticholinergics);
(b) Tardive dyskinesia;
(c) Hypothalamic side effects (amenorrhea, galactorrhea, appetite changes);
(d) Adrenolytic effects (orthostatic hypotension, drowsiness, nasal stuffiness, etc.);
(e) Seizures;
(f) Phototoxicity; and
(g) Organic psychosis

g) Antidepressants. These compounds are used for primary depression (usually endogenous), depression associated with hysteroid states, phobic anxiety, and eneuresis in children.

(1) They are classified as:

(a) Tricyclics (e.g., imipramine, amitriptyline, doxepin); and

(b) Monoamine oxidase inhibitors (MAOI's), (e.g., tranylcypromine)

(2) Procedures for their use are indicated below:

(a) Tricyclics must be administered for 1-3 weeks before they produce a clinical response. Start with a low dose tid, increasing every few days until a therapeutic response is achieved or until the maximum therapeutic levels permitted are reached. After 2-3 weeks, the drug may be given in a single daily dose hs. A drug with sedating side effects should be chosen if the patient is agitated.

(b) MAOI's have a narrow therapeutic range vis-a-vis their toxic range, and a given dose will often require 2-3 weeks of use before the side effects and therapeutic effects fully develop. Beginning with a dose at the low end of the therapeutic range, dosage is advanced every two weeks until response occurs or unacceptable side effects manifest.

(3) Side effects of the tricyclics include anticholinergic and andrenolytic effects. The MAOI's have no anticholinergic side effects, but increasing agitation and headache and potentially dangerous hypertensive episodes may result from excessive build-up of both endogenous amines and from exogenously administered sympathomimetic drugs and dietary tyramine. Special precautions, including attention to diet, are needed for all patients receiving MAOI's.

h) Lithium. Lithium is used for the treatment and/or prevention of manic episodes, as well as prevention of depressive episodes in manic-depressive patients. It may also be useful in the immediate treatment of depression in some manic-depressive patients and in controlling explosive outbursts of violence in certain types of character disorders.

(1) Procedures for its use should take note of the fact that therapeutic effects are associated with an optimal plasma lithium level which must be followed closely and adjusted by dosage change in the early phases of the therapy. Once stabilization has occurred, the frequency of plasma lithium determinations may be spaced out and decreased to a frequency of 1-3 months at maintenance levels. Some manic patients may require both lithium and antipsychotics. Because of the narrow range of

therapeutic efficacy and the closeness of that range to toxic levels, special care is important in the use of lithium.

(2) Side effects include:

(a) Gastrointestinal (e.g., nausea, vomiting, diarrhea);
(b) Nervous system effects (e.g., fine tremor, anergia, muscle weakness, slurred speech, confusion, muscle twitching, hyperpyrexia);
(c) Polyuria and polydipsia; and
(d) Toxicity occurs at levels of 2 mEq/L or less

i) Anti-anxiety drugs. These drugs are used for their anxiolytic and hypnotic effects. They are not antipsychotic in their effects, but are used for muscle relaxant and anticonvulsant effects. They are useful in alcohol withdrawal.

(1) The benzodiazepines include long- and short-acting types. The short-acting groups include oxazepam and lorazepam. The longer-acting groups include chloridazepoxide, diazepam and prazepam.

(2) Procedures for their use suggest that the short-acting drugs be administered in tid or qid doses, and the longer-acting drugs be administered bid or hs. Treatment should be limited to a few weeks rather than for many months. IM use is less effective in this class of drugs. In alcohol withdrawal, tapering the doses may facilitate detoxification. They may be used in combination with antidepressants for agitated depression, and are also used in some types of seizure disorder.

(3) Side effects feature an anergic CNS depression or paradoxical excitement and confusion, especially in the elderly. The major problem with these compounds is physical and psychological dependence.

7. Who treats?

a) Team responsibility or individual therapist responsibility? One basic premise of a CMHC is that the center assumes responsibility for providing mental health services to a total area population. This premise implies that direct treatment is the responsibility of the center and not that of a specific CMHC therapist to whom the patient may be assigned. Indeed, it is one of the strengths of the CMHC movement. Team or shared responsibility is supposed to provide a more thoughtful approach to the problems of any given patient and is supposed to provide sharing of the responsibility - especially in regard to night and weekend responsiveness. Team responsibility means that the patient can be provided whatever treatment is needed, and not just that particular treatment which the therapist alone can give. A larger group of seriously ill patients can be treated by a team than by an individual therapist because the pressures and demands of needy and disturbed individuals can be shared among team members. However, this team responsibility sometimes gives way to the "private practice model" - a model in which a variety of mental health professionals happen to practice under the roof of a CMHC. When the therapist begins to consider a CMHC patient as his personal patient, and when that therapist begins to insist upon making all the decisions relative to that patient's treatment, then this is more akin to solo practice than to team operation. The ideal CMHC is one in which several mental health professions are represented and are sharing responsibility for treatment planning and treatment implementation. In such a team, all members of the group feel responsible for all patients, even though a single member of that team may take the major responsibility for a given patient. Cases are reviewed at the time of treatment planning and periodically thereafter. This serves to review the utilization of therapeutic time and offers an approach to quality assurance of the treatment itself. It also provides a continuing education for members of the health team.

b) Skills of specific team members - generalist and specialist. The mental health team often consists of members of the four primary mental health professions: psychiatrists, clinical psychologists, clinical social workers and mental health nurses (usually at the clinical specialist level of training). The team is supplemented by the services of others, including administrators, paraprofessionals, adjunctive or activity therapists (occupational, recreational, art, music, etc.), and volunteers. Special counselors (drug, alcohol and vocational rehabilitation) are also found on mental health teams. There are clear differences in the practices of these professionals and paraprofessionals, as well as similarities. The similarities include a value system - a commitment to the community mental health model - as well as generalist skills in case evaluation and certain types of treatment. There will be major differences between the psychiatrist (a physician with 4-5 years of postmedical school training) and the paraprofessional, to name only two groups. However, all groups should have some cross-over skills and they should share a common approach in their efforts to understand patients and their families. They all should have some measure of skill in providing support and therapeutic help to the patients. (The false notion that any relationship which offers support and reassurance somehow constitutes psychotherapy is addressed in Section 5 on psychotherapy.) But every member of the team has a particular set of skills to be applied during some phase of psychotherapy. In addition to his generalist skills such as basic interviewing and assessment, each representative on the mental health team possesses skills unique to that particular profession. The psychiatrist who is a psychoanalyst will have had 8-10 years of training (usually half-time) _after_ his residency, and will have had more training and experience in doing exploratory psychotherapy than most other mental health specialists. The psychiatrist as a physician will have had broad training in medicine and the specialty of psychiatry. This gives him the background to evaluate the presence or absence of physical disease, the legal right and training to perform somatic methods of treatment and pharmacotherapy, to hospitalize, and to communicate effectively with other physicians. The clinical psychologist will have developed specialized skills in psychodiagnostic assessment, and in research design and statistical analysis. This does not obviate his skills as a clinician and as a consultant. The clinical social worker will have developed specialized knowledge about the community and its resources and will have accumulated experience in dealing with families and social service agencies. The mental health nurse-clinician will have knowledge of hospital and ambulatory treatment approaches and will have developed some specialized skills in hospital milieu.

Each profession has specific and well-defined training programs which are accredited by nationally recognized agencies. The accreditation focuses on the quality of the training program, and not on the individuals who are being trained. In psychiatry, the medical schools are accredited by the Liaison Committee on Medical Education (of the AMA and AAMC) while psychiatry residency programs are accredited by Residency Review Committees of the AMA, the American Board of Psychiatry & Neurology and the Accreditation Committee on Graduate Medical Education. The accreditation of approved doctoral training programs in clinical psychology is done by the American Psychological Association.

Certification and licensure of individuals as specialists is done by other groups. In psychiatry, such certification is carried on by the American Board of Psychiatry & Neurology. Licensure is yet another procedure and is done by state-level bodies who grant the legal right to carry on a defined practice. Psychologists are licensed in many states; and psychiatrists are licensed as physicians in all states. Other professions have their own accreditation, certification and licensure procedures. Some are not credentialed in the same manner from state to state, and many are seeking procedures for standardizing the credentialing process - both to protect the public and to improve their own professions.

c) <u>Consultation and supervision.</u> Despite the outstanding benefits of team orientation, many CMHC personnel choose to follow the individual practice model. Indeed, many have left the center after gaining some experience in order to acquire the (presumed) autonomy and financial rewards of private practice. Nevertheless, quality professional practice in a

CMHC calls for shared responsibility and each member of the team should have regular consultation with or supervision by another mental health professional. Regardless of whether that person is a member of the same profession or another profession, the key issues are guidance and education. The consultant or supervisor should have a level of competence, knowledge and communicative skills sufficient to enhance continuously the knowledge base and performance of the consultee or supervisee. The term "consultation" is often preferred in place of "supervision", as the latter is sometimes construed to mean having administrative control or authority over the supervisee. Actually, the term "supervision" comes from psychiatric training, wherein the supervisor is a teacher and consultant, rather than a "boss". But semantics are not without their emotional determinants, and the major concern is that the professional member be given ample opportunity to discuss the treatment of a given family, patient or group with another skilled person. This process enables the consultee to learn more about the treatment itself, and can also provide a sounding board for the therapist who may be experiencing emotional problems generated by the therapeutic situation.

d) Medical "back-up". The patients who come to a CMHC are entitled to the highest quality service which can be arranged. This means that attention must be paid to their biological, psychological and social needs. Physical illness often mimics the symptoms of mental disorder, and a number of studies have shown that some patients in CMHC's who present with mental symptoms are actually suffering from physical disease. The mental disorder of these patients clears when the physical disease is treated. Attention should be given to the physical condition of every patient, whether hospitalized or treated in an ambulatory setting; and there should be proof of a recent (no more than 3-6 months previous) physical examination, together with appropriate laboratory tests or other diagnostic procedures (x-rays, EKG or other tests) in the record. The physical exam may be performed by a member of the CMHC medical staff or by another physician in the community whose report is then entered in the patient's file. The patient should be given the best treatment possible for the given condition(s) he brings. This could involve somatic-pharmacotherapy or ECT. It could also mean hospitalization. None of these caveats are meant to suggest that every patient should be treated only by a psychiatrist. But they do mean that a psychiatrist should be involved in the evaluation and treatment planning of every patient if that patient is to be given full access to the special medical skills and overall knowledge of bio-psycho-social aspects of behavior known to the psychiatrist. It also means that a psychiatrist or other physician should be available to the nonmedical therapist during the ongoing treatment - not for the purpose of controlling the treatment or supervising the psychotherapy, but rather, to determine whether the patient could be developing some hitherto unsuspected organic disease, or if the patient's condition develops in such a way as to indicate somatic treatment. Sometimes it is in the patient's best interest to have a medication program added to the psychotherapy already in progress. In some of the current struggles over turf and control, the patient's needs have been overlooked.

8. Treatment-management of special conditions

a) Schizophrenia. Patients with a diagnosis of schizophrenia constitute one of the largest populations treated in a CMHC. Because of the chronicity of this condition, these patients require attention for many years after the disorder first comes to the attention of the center staff. Recent changes in the diagnostic manual (DSM III) have improved the criteria and enhanced the precision with which this diagnosis is made. Although schizophrenics once constituted a large proportion of patients in state mental hospitals, the arrival of antipsychotic medications and community treatment approaches have made it possible for many of these patients to be treated in the community - at least for most phases of the disorder.

(1) Diagnosis.* The patient must display at least one of the following during a phase of the illness:

*Diagnostic criteria are from the new DSM III

(a) Bizarre delusions (content is patently absurd and has no possible basis in fact) such as delusions of being controlled, thought broadcasting, thought insertion, or thought withdrawal;

(b) Somatic, grandiose, religious, nihilistic, or other delusions without persecutory or jealous content;

(c) Delusions with persecutory or jealous content if accompanied by hallucinations of any type;

(d) Auditory hallucinations in which either a voice keeps up a running commentary on the individual's behavior or thoughts, or two or more voices are conversing with each other;

(e) Auditory hallucinations on several occasions, with content of more than one or two words having no apparent relation to depression or elation; and/or

(f) Incoherence, marked loosening of associations, markedly illogical thinking, or marked poverty of content of speech if associated with at least one of the following:

(1) Blunted, flat or inappropriate affect;
(2) Delusions or hallucinations; and/or
(3) Catatonic or other grossly disorganized behavior

There must be deterioration from a previous level of functioning in such areas as work, social relations or self-care. There must be continuous signs of the illness for a period of at least six months during the person's life, with some signs of the illness presently in view. (See DSM III for definitions of the prodromal phase, the residual phase and prodromal or residual symptoms.) If a full depressive or manic syndrome is present, it either developed after the psychotic symptoms or was brief in duration relative to the duration of the psychotic symptoms previously listed. The onset of the prodromal or active phase of the illness must have occurred before age 45, and it must not be due to any organic mental disorder or mental retardation.

(2) Prognosis or course of illness. There is a wide range of manifestations of this disorder - some are acute and brief and do not persist, while in others there is a slowly deteriorating course. Indicators of good prognosis include:

(a) Acute onset with tension and anxiety as well as verbal aggression;
(b) Good premorbid social and work history;
(c) Depressive symptoms and concern with guilt and death;
(d) Clear precipitating factors;
(e) Family history of affective disorder and no such history of schizophrenia; and
(f) The patient has been married

Indicators of poor prognosis include:

(a) Insidious onset with withdrawn behavior and emotional blunting;
(b) Little overt hostility but clear sensorium;
(c) Excessive persecutory delusions and paranoia;
(d) Schizoid or asocial premorbid personality; and
(e) Family history of schizophrenia and absence of affective symptoms

(3) Treatment of the acute schizophrenic

(a) Hospitalization may or may not be indicated depending upon the motivation of the patient, the presence of a social support system which is cooperative, the degree of potential danger to self or others, etc. (see Section 4 on hospitalization). Some acute schizophrenics can be treated without hospitalization if the circumstances are favorable. Many, however, are hospitalized for a brief period - perhaps 2-4 weeks. That general length of stay has frequently been found necessary to achieve compensation and to plan for the outpatient phase of treatment.

(b) Medications are frequently (almost always) used in treating psychotic symptoms. The antipsychotics are indicated in conjunction with any necessary compounds for modifying undesirable side effects (see Section 6 on pharmacotherapy).

(c) Psychotherapy is begun at this phase (if the patient is not yet in treatment) and the hospitalization is often an opportunity to establish a therapeutic alliance and institute psychotherapy. If at all possible, the patient should be assigned to a therapist who can treat the patient in all phases of the illness and in both the hospital and outpatient clinic settings. Continuity of care is especially important since extended chronicity may develop and because the downward course often associated with schizophrenia may be altered by a singular long-term psychotherapeutic relationship. Psychotherapy is generally supportive, with cautious exploration into the precipitating events of the acute illness. Insight-oriented psychotherapy or intensive and regressive maneuvers are generally not used, though a few highly experienced therapists advocate such an approach.

(d) The family is an important consideration. Their cooperation must be enlisted in treatment and long-term management. In many programs family psychotherapy is considered the basic approach to treatment. There is much evidence of family psychopathology and shared systems of paralogical cognitive processes which may be influenced by family therapy.

(4) Treatment of the chronic schizophrenic requires additional planning and recognition of the necessity for a rehabilitation-resocialization approach. The chronic schizophrenic is often one who has been a patient in a state mental hospital for one or more prolonged periods of time. Management in the community requires attention to residential treatment with gradations in the movement from supervised living to unsupervised settings. The patient is likely to be on maintenance medication for years - some would say for life. This requires careful management in order to avoid neurologic complications such as tardive dyskinesia (see Section 6 on pharmacotherapy). Chronic schizophrenics do best when they remain in contact with one therapist who will be available for long periods of time - several years, generally. The therapist (if not a physician) must have medical support and backup to manage the medication. Since these patients are often treated in multi-agency settings and because they sometimes depend on public welfare programs for financial support, the "case manager" concept came into being. The case manager is a mental health professional or paraprofessional who is responsible for the coordination of various services needed during community maintenance and rehabilitation of the chronic schizophrenic. It is especially important that the case manager be responsible for aggressive and continuous follow-up. At various times in their illness these patients may require partial hospitalization, brief periods of acute hospitalization and, possibly, periods of less intensive treatment in 24-hour care centers. Crisis intervention is always an important resource in the community management of such patients.

b) Affective disorders. These patients may suffer from bipolar or unipolar manic-depressive disease or from depressive neuroses (dysthymic disorders).

(1) Manic episodes are defined as one or more distinct periods of a predominantly elevated, expansive or irritable mood exhibited by the

patient. The elevated or irritable mood must be a prominent part of the illness and relatively persistent, although it may alternate or intermingle with a depressive mood. The duration must be for at least one week (or any duration, if hospitalization becomes necessary) during which at least three of the following symptoms have persisted most of the time (four if the mood is only irritable) and to a significant degree:

(a) Increase in activity (either socially, at work or sexually) or physical restlessness;

(b) More talkative than usual or pressure to keep talking;

(c) Flight of ideas or subjective experience that thoughts are racing;

(d) Inflated self-esteem (grandiosity, which may be delusional);

(e) Decreased need for sleep;

(f) Distractibility, i.e., attention too easily drawn to unimportant or irrelevant external stimuli; or

(g) Excessive involvement in activities that have a high potential for painful consequences which are not recognized - e.g., buying sprees, sexual indiscretions, foolish business investments, reckless driving

There should be no clear evidence of schizophrenia, organic mental disorder or preoccupation with mood-incongruent delusions or hallucinations or bizarre behavior (see DSM III for definitions of mood-congruent and incongruent psychotic features).

(2) Major depressive episodes are defined as a dysphoric mood or loss of interest in all or almost all usual activities or pastimes exhibited

by the patient. The dysphoric mood is characterized by symptomatic descriptions such as: "depressed," "sad," "blue," "hopeless," "low," "down in the dumps," "irritable." The mood disturbance must be prominent and relatively persistent, but not necessarily the most dominant symptom. Momentary shifts from one dysphoric mood to another (e.g., from anxiety to depression to anger) are not to be counted in measuring persistence. At least four of the following symptoms must have been present collectively for a period of at least 14 consecutive days:

(a) Poor appetite or significant weight loss (when not dieting) or increased appetite or significant weight gain;

(b) Insomnia or hypersomnia;

(c) Psychomotor agitation or retardation (but not merely subjective feelings of restlessness or being slowed down);

(d) Loss of interest or pleasure in usual activities, or decrease in sexual drive not limited to a period when delusional or hallucinating;

(e) Loss of energy, fatigue;

(f) Feelings of worthlessness, self-reproach, or excessive or inappropriate guilt (either may be delusional);

(g) Complaints or evidence of diminished ability to think or concentrate, such as slowed thinking, or indecisiveness not associated with marked loosening of associations or incoherence; and

(h) Recurrent thoughts of death, suicidal ideation, death wishes, or a suicide attempt

There should be no clear evidence of schizophrenia, organic mental disorder or preoccupation with a mood-incongruent delusion or hallucination or bizarre behavior.

(3) Depressive neurosis (or dysthymic disorder) is defined as requiring that during the past two years (or one year for children and adolescents) the individual has been bothered most or all of the time by symptoms characteristic of the depressive syndrome. These symptoms should not be of sufficient severity and duration to meet the criteria for a major depressive disorder. The manifestations may be relatively persistent or separated by periods of normal mood lasting a few days to a few weeks, but no more than a few months at a time. During the depressive periods, there is either a prominent depressed mood (e.g., sad, blue, down in the dumps, low) or marked loss of interest or pleasure in almost all usual activities and pastimes. During the depressive periods, at least three of the following symptoms must be present:

(a) Insomnia or hypersomnia;
(b) Low energy level or chronic tiredness;
(c) Feelings of inadequacy, loss of self-esteem or self-deprecation;
(d) Decreased effectiveness or productivity at school, work or home;
(e) Decreased attention, concentration, or ability to think clearly;
(f) Social withdrawal;
(g) Loss of interest in or enjoyment of pleasurable activities;
(h) Irritability or excessive anger;
(i) Inability to respond with apparent pleasure to praise or rewards;
(j) Less active or talkative than usual, or feels slowed down or restless;
(k) Pessimistic attitude toward the future, brooding about past events, or feeling sorry for self;
(l) Tearfulness or crying; and
(m) Recurrent thoughts of death or suicide

There should be no psychotic features such as delusions or hallucinations.

(4) Prognosis or course of illness. True manic-depressive disease is by definition one which is likely to recur. Neurotic depressions are

not periodic in character, but are persistent over months and/or years. The major problem with the depressive illness is the risk of suicide. Suicide risk may be evaluated by considering the following factors:

(a) History of prior attempt: approximately 40% of suicides have tried before;

(b) Occupation: the unemployed have higher suicide rates. Suicide is higher in areas of employment such as police work, medicine and certain other professions;

(c) Marital status: single persons are at a greater risk;

(d) Sex: men commit suicide three times as often as women. The unemployed middle-aged man with a recent life crisis, such as a health problem or the recent loss of a loved one, and who uses alcohol is probably at highest risk;

(e) Age: more frequent in older men and in women under 60. Suicide among adolescents is increasing;

(f) Family history: the higher the incidence of suicide in the family, the higher the lethality;

(g) Emotional factors: depression, psychosis, alcoholism are all high-risk states; and

(h) Health: recent serious illness with loss of hope is a special risk factor

(5) Treatment may or may not involve hospitalization. The assessment of suicide risk is of special importance in deciding whether to hospitalize the patient or not. The other factor to be assessed is the social support system. Even a seriously depressed patient can be treated outside the hospital if there is an ideal support system and someone who can stay with

the patient constantly. Medication is the first approach (the antidepressants), in coordination with psychotherapy. Few therapists would advocate the use of psychotherapy without antidepressants. After a trial of antidepressants (at least two), if there is no response, ECT should be considered. For the depressive neurosis (dysthymic disorder), ECT has not generally been advocated. Psychotherapy is the treatment of choice, with or without antidepressants. For manic reactions, lithium is the treatment generally used first. If there is not a prompt response, the clinician will generally shift to either antipsychotics or to ECT. For the wildly excited manic who has a truly life-threatening illness, ECT may be life-saving. After the manic attack has subsided, the patient should be placed on lithium for prophylaxis. Some feel that lithium prevents further depressive episodes.

c) Organic brain syndromes involve alteration (temporary or permanent) of brain function. It may have a variety of causes. DSM III identifies and categorizes the organic brain syndromes as: delirium and dementia, organic hallucinosis, organic delusional or affective syndromes, intoxication, and other types. Delirium is a rapidly developing and fluctuating disorder marked by a disturbance of attention. Dementia is a deterioration of intellectual capacity which is sufficient to impair the patient's functioning.

(1) Diagnosis of delirium. There is clouding of consciousness (reduced clarity of awareness of the environment) with reduced capacity to shift, focus and sustain attention to environmental stimuli. There must be at least two of the following symptoms exhibited:

(a) Perceptual disturbance (misinterpretations, illusions or hallucinations);
(b) Speech that is sometimes incoherent;
(c) Disturbance of a sleep-wakefulness cycle with insomnia or daytime drowsiness; and
(d) Increased or decreased psychomotor activity

Disorientation and memory impairment must be present. The clinical features develop over a short period of time (hours to days) and tend to fluctuate over the course of a day. There should be evidence from history, physical examination or laboratory tests of a specific organic factor deemed to be etiologically related to this disorder.

(2) Diagnosis of dementia. There is loss of intellectual abilities of sufficient severity to interfere with social or occupational functioning. Memory impairment is present along with at least one of the following:

(a) Impairment of abstract thinking, as manifested by concrete interpretation of proverbs, inability to find similarities and differences between related words, difficulty in defining words and concepts and other similar tasks;

(b) Impaired judgment;

(c) Other disturbances of higher cortical function, such as aphasia (disorder of language due to brain dysfunction), apraxia (inability to carry out motor activities despite intact comprehension), agnosia (failure to recognize or identify objects despite intact sensory function), constructional difficulty (inability to copy three-dimensional figures, assemble blocks or arrange sticks in specific designs); or

(d) Personality change, i.e., alteration or accentuation of premorbid traits

Consciousness should not be clouded as in delirium or intoxication. There should be evidence of a specific organic factor judged to be etiologically related to the disturbance. If the evidence is absent, an organic factor can be presumed if conditions other than organic mental disorders have been reasonably excluded, and the behavioral change represents cognitive impairment in a variety of areas. It should be noted that "dementia" as used above is not deemed to be irreversible, which was the way this term used to be defined.

(3) Diagnosis of amnesic syndrome calls for:

(a) Both short-term and long-term memory impairment;

(b) No clouding of consciousness (as in delirium or intoxication) or general loss of major intellectual abilities (as in dementia); and

(c) Evidence of a specific organic cause of the disturbance

(4) Diagnosis of organic delusional syndrome calls for:

(a) Delusions are the predominant clinical feature;

(b) No clouding of consciousness, significant loss of intellectual abilities or prominent hallucinations; and

(c) Evidence of a specific organic cause of the disturbance

(5) Diagnosis of organic hallucinosis calls for:

(a) Persistent or recurrent hallucinations as the predominant clinical feature;

(b) No clouding of consciousness, significant intellectual ability loss, predominant delusions or predominant mood disturbance; and

(c) Evidence of a specific organic cause of the disturbance

(6) Diagnosis of organic personality syndrome calls for:

(a) Marked change in behavior or personality involving at least one of the following:

(1) Emotional lability (e.g., explosive temper, sudden crying);
(2) Impairment in impulse control (e.g., poor judgment, sexual indiscretions, shoplifting);
(3) Marked apathy and indifference; and/or
(4) Suspiciousness or paranoid ideation

(b) There should be no clouding of consciousness, significant loss of intellectual abilities, predominant mood disturbance, predominant delusions or hallucinations.

(c) Evidence of a specific organic cause of the disturbance must be present.

(7) Diagnosis of intoxication calls for:

(a) Development of substance-specific syndrome following recent ingestion and measurable presence in the body of an intoxicating substance;

(b) Maladaptive behavior during waking state due to effect of substance on CNS (e.g., impaired judgment, belligerence); and

(c) Clinical features which do not correspond to other specific organic brain syndromes

(8) Treatment or management will depend on the specific etiology of the organic brain syndrome. General management should include establishment of a comforting and familiar environment. Sedatives should be avoided. Agitated, psychotic patients would benefit from small doses of antipsychotic drugs.

CHAPTER 5

TREATMENT OF CHILDREN AND FAMILIES IN COMMUNITY MENTAL HEALTH CENTERS

Irving N. Berlin, M.D.

1. Diagnosis and evaluation

   a) Population to be served and primary care aspects of evaluation:

      (1) All elements of population served by law; lower socioeconomic class mostly served because of service availability and referral.

      (2) All children require physical examinations and a thorough evaluation of health history and current medical problems.

      (3) School populations referred by schools because of learning and behavior problems are most frequent clients seen. These populations require:

         (a) Total evaluation of health records, illnesses, recent medical work-ups, and arrangements for pediatric examinations and immunizations

(b) Work with parents who may be obliged to come to the school in order to keep the child in school; need special techniques to involve alienated parents in evaluation

(c) Special evaluation processes in the case of children who will not talk easily

(4) Adolescents with behavior problems and problems associated with drugs and antisocial acting out (often court referred) require:

(a) Medical evaluation for special problems - vision, hearing, diabetes, or other illness

(b) Special work with parents who have often given up

(5) Children from disorganized families (parents with major problems in living, finding work, relating to each other, keeping finances straight, and who harbor anger at agencies or at demands of children) which include:

(a) Abused and neglected children

(b) Children with severe, chronic psychophysiologic illness

(c) Children with severe learning and behavior problems in preschool and elementary school

(d) Children showing withdrawal and isolated behavior, fear of adults and children

(6) Preschool children with problems permitting early intervention and prevention. These problems may require:

(a) Child development and parenting classes to help mothers particularly to deal with young children

(b) Stimulation play groups to facilitate the development of the child's autonomy, curiosity, playfulness and capacity to relate to adults and other children

(c) Home visits to help parents with new interactions with young child

(7) High-risk infants and young children. Development-stimulation clinics may be useful in:

(a) Teaching parents methods of observing and stimulating babies and young children

(b) Making specific developmental diagnoses and providing stimulation programs for each child

(c) Establishing no future goals for each mother-infant pair over 1-3-month periods

(d) Enabling parents to work with other babies in infant development classes to learn how to help other infants and to develop capacities in new mothers; home visits to new mothers may encourage their participation

(8) Children with acute and chronic developmental handicaps such as mental retardation. Their progress should be reassessed and help provided:

(a) To parents to accept the child's handicap or limitations

(b) To parents to talk with the child through demonstrations

(c) To consider the needs of other family members

(d) To reduce difficult attention-demanding behaviors which disturb family life and affect the child's capacity for maximal adaptive living and learning

b) Purposes of evaluation:

(1) Assessment of problems in terms of a complaint about the child related to:

(a) Child's developmental stage and deviations

(b) Family needs and place of child in family

(c) Social systems surrounding child and their impact on child and family

(2) Assessment of the adaptive strengths of the child; that is, the developmental assessment of the child's psychosocial, cognitive, physical-social adaptive strengths

(3) Assessment of the adaptive and coping strengths of the family, including the family's capacity:

(a) To work;
(b) To manage money;
(c) To keep itself together with most children functioning;
(d) To deal with the illness of family members; and
(e) To deal with community agencies effectively

(4) Careful developmental assessment of the identified patient, including:

(a) Cognitive, psychosocial-physical and social-interactional aspects to identify the developmental level attained in each area

(b) Psychopathological factors and their implications for ego development, using the Erikson-White scales of ego deficits

(5) Diagnosis using a multiaxial approach for both child and family

(6) Determination of modalities of treatment that would be most effective in dealing with problems.

(7) Determination of goals of treatment for all persons involved

(8) Statement of prognosis under ideal conditions, depending on:

(a) Involvement of parents

(b) Involvement of schools and other agencies
(c) Availability of skilled therapists in most relevant treatment modality

(9) Statement of prognosis under current conditions of therapeutic engagement:

(a) What are the outcome measures of effective treatment with child? with parents?

(b) Could the involvement of parents or agencies be increased?

(10) Prediction of length of treatment process to achieve realistic goals

(11) Statement of when progress needs to be reviewed. Consideration should be given to:

(a) Assessment of goals and treatment modalities in the light of experience.

(b) Alteration of modalities, goals-prognosis-outcome expectation or duration of treatment:

(1) When will the case be next reviewed?
(2) Should it be reviewed with the family?

c) Special evaluation processes:

(1) Group evaluations with brief 15-20 minute individual contacts with parents and with child presenting problems. Signed permission should be obtained for group evaluations.

(a) An evaluation worker should help families to fill out medical and parent questionnaires. Special questions should be discussed aloud, as well as the reasons for these questions being asked and their importance.

(b) The evaluation worker should explain how financial liability is assessed and how it will be done individually, with a focus on the usual concerns of parents and the kinds of questions often unasked.

(c) The evaluation worker should focus on the similarity of problems with children that brings families here with a discussion of:

(1) The expectations schools have of children;

(2) Parents' questions and concerns regarding the schools; and

(3) Parents' understanding of the teachers' and principals' interests and concerns with children

(a) Learning problems and their meanings

(b) How had each parent done in school

(d) The worker may assume the role of child advocate and talk about how children often feel in school. Children have their own sense of what is unfair in demands made on them to learn. The worker tries to elicit the child's comments and agreement of children about the kinds of problems they find in school.

(e) The worker helps parents to see how important they are to their children and their learning process.

(1) The worker should help parents recall how they felt when their own parents did or did not care about their school success or failure, did or did not inquire about their school and learning activities.

(2) What are the parents' aspirations for their children?

(3) School visits by parents may help the parents with problems and possible solutions.

(4) Community workers should help in assessments.

(2) Use of evaluation to help parents understand why their continued involvement is important.

(a) Use of evaluation group to move into parent group to teach them how to help their children to learn, even when they do not remember much about math, etc.

(1) Use of Bereiter-Engelman parent-learning techniques

(2) Use of Parent Effectiveness Training method of rewards from parents for child's effective learning

(3) Home visit evaluations with families whose children are troubled in school and who have difficulty coming to clinic.

(a) Use of familiar setting to explore not only child's problems but family's concerns in general

(b) Beginning of family effort to consider problems in living by use of assessment tools; parents, family and individual health questionnaires to find various foci of troubles as family is helped to fill out these questionnaires

(c) Developmentally trained mental health professionals and paraprofessionals should use functioning of child in home to assess development and developmental needs; similar assessments of developmental status of other children in family

(d) Evaluation of how family views community agencies and of their capacity to use these agencies effectively; what are obstacles to such use?

(e) Use of home evaluation to determine location of ongoing therapeutic work if assessment shows need. Possible work in the home could be a beginning of family involvement in problem-solving.

(4) Mental health workers may involve the family and child and meet with the school or another agency to:

(a) Understand problems better;

(b) Understand how parents can help;

(c) Help parents express their feelings about the school and their needs from school. For example, a child may be absent from school but the parents are never informed; a child may be disciplined for trouble in school but parents are not involved in understanding the problem;

(d) Make known to the school the family's current stresses or problems so that the school may be aware of them;

(e) Develop a plan for communication between the family and school involving mental health worker; and

(f) Help the family to take advantage of the school's programs to assist parents

(1) Parent education and parenting programs

(2) Parent-child activity programs

(a) Worker may need to come with family until they feel engaged in the alien-feeling school

(b) Worker may need to find school person with skills to relate to family and keep in touch with them

(5) Assessments may have to be done over time by developmentally trained workers in:

(a) The home, as previously described

(b) Preschool-school, to get an idea of behaviors under social and learning conditions

(c) Foster or other family settings, such as visits to foster homes, receiving facility, court, etc. when invited or when necessary to understand particular "parental" behavior in a particular setting

(6) Assessment and evaluation conferences may review the purpose of assessments as indicated in the section on the purpose of evaluation, in order to:

(a) Develop plans for treatment

(b) Develop plans for regular assessment and review of treatment and evaluation of conclusions

(c) Make plans for possible discharge date, agencies to be involved, future evaluation

d) Evaluation is made of a variety of children's problems:

(1) Neurotic problems and behavior problems related to fears, obsessive and compulsive behavior, or nightmares

(2) Learning problems related to internalized neurotic problems, failure to develop curiosity and capacity for learning due to deprivations and maladaptive educative methods or personnel

(3) Organic problems as elicited by a history of prenatal, birth or postnatal problems:

(a) Minimal brain dysfunction with short attention span, hyperactive behavior and incapacity to learn, with a history of birth trauma and early onset of hypermotility and disturbed rhythms of sleep and feeding

(b) Autism with family history and clear signs of vestibular and midbrain disturbances

(c) Mental retardation - especially mild and moderate retardation - with accompanying psychological problems related to child's failures as compared to peers

(d) Metabolic problems - like phenylketonuria (P. K. U) - which may require help to a child already diagnosed with adaptive functioning

(e) Perceptual-motor problems which may require diagnostic evaluation in collaboration with a school specialist, and help with the accompanying motivational and emotional problems

e) Intrafamilial problems, which include:

(1) Neurotic problems:

(a) School phobia is an example where the needs of the parent to keep a child near for his or her own comfort bring about fears in a child that the parent will die, etc. if the child is in school.

(2) Psychotic problems:

(a) History of maternal depression, gross deprivation and developmental failure in child

(b) Childhood psychosis. There is a need to examine the degree to which parental and family problems contribute to the child's difficulties

(3) Psychophysiologic problems; these require a review of family understanding of any illness: how they handle episodes, or how much independence/dependence becomes a problem.

(a) Asthma

(b) Gastrointestinal problems

(c) Diabetes. Additional problems may be brought on by separation, divorce or death of one parent with an overload on the other parent.

(d) Anorexia nervosa. This is the most likely psychosis and often the most chronically life-threatening. History of early feeding concerns should be taken.

(4) Learning and behavior problems; must be evaluated in the context of family problems in a culture which does or does not facilitate learning.

(a) Non-concern of family regarding education may be a primary source of the child's lack of concern with learning. The failure to learn leads to behavior problems and the need to determine sequences of problems - at what age and grade they occurred - to understand the etiology

(b) Family problems with disorganized families

(1) Alcoholism - care of child is highly variable with a high potential for abuse and neglect

(2) Drug addiction - as above, with increased periods of parents' lack of awareness of infants' signals and needs, resulting in marked deprivation

(5) Child abuse and neglect may be detected from repeated histories of injuries and failure to thrive nutritionally.

(a) Parental history of abuse and neglect and tendencies to impulsive behavior and projection on others of own failures, hurt and anger

(b) Lack of parental models in parents' own development; no clear expectations and practice in helping children to grow up

(c) Expectations that child behave like an adult, inability to nurture child and enjoy child, with consequent crying and disturbing behavior of child

f) Multiaxial developmental diagnosis to permit total evaluation:

(1) Cognitive development:

(a) I.Q. -culturally corrected and linked to capacities for learning

(b) Cognitive levels of functioning as examined for in Piaget's testing methods

(2) Socio-cultural factors. Expectations of child in culture, role of child in family and expectations for being a miniature adult or baby

(3) Interpersonal psychodynamic development - ego psychology: evaluation of ego development in Erikson's schemata and psychosexual levels

of development and maldevelopment. Statement of levels of fixation or regression in terms of failures to develop or reactions to stress with loss of adaptive capacities

(4) Neurophysiologic development: attainment of developmental milestones

(5) Psychopathologic experiences which interfere with development: early deprivation, parental loss at a particular stage of development, incest, abuse, etc.

g) Evaluation may be used to determine intervention and modalities of treatment as well as who should be involved:

(1) Diagnosis should carry a statement about prognosis with ideal treatment modality and probabilities of success with modalities available.

(2) Developmental evaluation provides milestones to be reached in each diagnostic axis in treatment.

(3) Probable duration of treatment should be noted for the purpose of further treatment evaluation research.

h) Evaluation must include a gross developmental diagnosis, a determination of the state of ego capacities and the degree of psychopathology of each parent.

2. Modalities of treatment. General issues: In community mental health centers the individual therapy of children, while often the only one therapists are trained for, ignores the developmental needs of children in favor of play socialization and group experience. There is a tendency not to look carefully at the possible therapeutic help available in the school and through the educational process.

a) Individual psychotherapy for child and adolescent:

(1) It is thought that young neurotic children without serious ego deficits can best utilize play therapy as a mode of communication of conflicts through the playing-out of fantasies and reacting favorably to interpretative behavior or comments

(2) Adolescents who need help with individuation and separation from family and have no gross reality deficits

(3) Other children from disorganized families where the family may not involve themselves in the treatment and who require a period of individual attention and reparenting prior to being able to function in groups

b) Child and parents in simultaneous collaborative treatment or conjoint counseling:

(1) One therapist sees child and parents in play or talking therapy so that all the facts from the history in evaluation and during course of treatment may be integrated, as well as having all treatment problems dealt with by one person (simultaneous therapeutic involvement).

(a) Risks about keeping confidentiality of child and parents in therapeutic work. Continued opportunities to demonstrate to child and parents that cross-communication does not occur. Only agreed-on topics and information are exchanged. Information is shared by all.

(2) One therapist works with the child alone with parents in couples treatment. This is often helpful with a neurotic or not very severe behavior problem which reflects exacerbation of marital problems. It is usually time limited.

(3) Collaboration of child's therapist with the therapist who sees each parent or both parents together may help children and parents who need exclusive professional therapy because of severe developmental problems in each.

(4) Indications for conjoint counseling: communication difficulties in family and family's tendency to divide authority and create turmoil. Child and each parent change allegiances which create and maintain problems between child and parents; frequent problems with authority in school; child and each parent may

present different views to school personnel; very time limited effort; collaboration is too difficult in this situation.

(5) Indications for collaborative treatment: when parents and child both desire resolution of conflicts and problems, when the family is well integrated and functions well in most areas, and when parents and child are developmentally sophisticated so they can use problem-solving techniques.

c) Conjoint family therapy is used when essential problems are intrafamilial:

(1) The disorder in the child is related to poor or distorted communications, or

(2) The child's role in family drama produces pathology and dysfunction for the child which cannot be altered without altering family behavior:

(a) Problems which involve a school-age child able to speak for himself and to parents. Exploration of role expectations, actual behaviors, adaptive and maladaptive communications, clarification of parental needs of child, parental models for each parent from own childhood, and task or problem-oriented effort to alter parenting behaviors and child's pathologic behaviors.

(b) Problems of a psychophysiologic nature like anorexia nervosa where early and severe family miscommunication and role assignment of sick child seriously hamper development and facilitate somatic expression of conflict. Requires prolonged clarification and task-oriented efforts to alter roles - assertive role of family therapist.

(c) School phobias where symbiosis of parents and child needs to be reduced by clarification of the developmental needs of child. Parents should be helped to find alternative gratifications in living.

(d) Problems in latency, age-distortions of oedipal problems with fears of own sexuality resulting in expectation of violent retaliation or desertion. The capacity to relate with adults and peers interferes with learning and social development due to neurotic fear.

 (1) Parents are amenable to examining their attitudes.

(e) Early and midadolescent problems:

 (1) Related to individuation, separation and learning to function as an adult; family unable to handle rebellion, set limits and to recognize requests for both nurturance and independence

  (a) Parents concerned with the struggle and desire to help with the adolescent's difficulties and the crises which often occur at this stage of development

  (b) Adolescent capable of talking about troubles with parents-previous history of good communication

 (2) Need for additional role models and assistance to family with very rigid authoritarian standards to help resolve struggle where previously the child had done well in school and socially

 (3) Sudden decompensation in adolescence due to sexual conflicts with good premorbid history - family unable to understand and cope - withdrawal and onset of mild phobias

(4) School phobia in adolescents as a sign of sexual anxieties and role identity requires support and help with socialization

(5) Suicidal behavior - help to family to look at possible messages and translate parental and adolescent behavior to each other with efforts to re-establish communications and to deal with conflicts openly and nondestructively - will not be as easy with psychotic individuals, i.e., suicide attempts

(6) Schizophrenic reaction of young adolescents with parents involved in long-term resolution of problems of individuation and their supportive role and providing new models

(f) Late adolescent problems:

(1) Sudden onset of severe withdrawal or learning problems, suicidal or hostile aggressive behavior where:

(a) Adolescent has not been able to separate from family

(b) Adolescent remains dependent on family and is unable to make other social relationships or sexual attachments

(2) Psychotic reactions of late adolescence with double bind situations with one or both parents requiring resolution

(3) Severe depressive or manic-depressive reactions where psychopharmacologic methods are only temporarily effective - all require

long-term working through of unresolved family conflicts and developing new relationships, models and communication patterns

3. Use of crisis situation to mobilize energies usually not available when defenses are up.

a) Crisis intervention:

(1) The crisis situation permits the following questions to be raised:

(a) What is the crisis? What precipitated it?
(b) Whom does it affect?
(c) Why is it disorganizing?
(d) What are the child's and family's resources for coping without intervention?

(2) The issues related to the crisis can be opened for discussion if the therapist is attuned to the unspoken issues and raises these as tentative possibilities.

(3) Assessment of individual and family ego strengths or coping abilities is important.

(4) The specific crisis, be it suicide, a psychosomatic crisis like diabetic coma, behavioral problems like rage, murderous threats, or school phobia, contains developmental and psychopathologic elements that need to be assessed and described.

(a) Example: A suicide attempt of a young adolescent has a different developmental and psychopathologic meaning from an attempt in a seven to eight-year-old child.

(5) A discussion of covert issues not at first discussed allows an analysis of the covert participants who may act behind the scenes to precipitate or permit a crisis through non-support and action in concert with the most anxious and involved parent.

(6) Re-examination of why the crisis occurs now may lead to a different understanding from the initial discussion since the process of problem-solving has started.

4. <u>Use of crisis theory to evaluate and intervene in a crisis.</u>

a) Theory states that in a crisis there is an optimal time during which changes can occur if mobilized energy is utilized; otherwise after several weeks, crisis leads to a shoring up of defenses and increases the rigidity of the defensive armor in all involved.

b) Crisis theory requires a major active role of the therapist to define tasks and help with the assessment of results:

(1) Example: Crisis of preadolescent or adolescent suicide allows family involvement in crisis treatment if terms are made prior to admission of adolescent to ward, otherwise crisis is given to the hospital to solve.

c) Use of precipitating cause of crisis as the focus of the intervention rather than underlying problems.

5. <u>Use of family supports</u>, i.e., help to family with extra child, etc., to cope with regular functions of family so more attention can be given to crisis solution.

a) Home help to mother with crisis of premature infant

b) Help with other children or elders to allow more time in hospital for family to work on crisis

6. <u>Use of task-oriented approach to crisis resolution.</u>

a) Requires specific behavioral interaction of each family member designed to help communication between family members to encourage more positive relations between persons most in conflict.

b) Example: A 12-year-old boy who stole a car and guns, and committed arson until apprehended. Discussion should clarify feelings about mother's going to work, father's anger with mother and his isolation from son and home. Previous support by father in sports and learning is gone; mother is angry at all men. Tasks for father may be to teach son to drive three times a week at a specified time. Mother to help son clean messy room she nags about. Mother and father to talk with therapist about meaning of mother's job, problems in home, etc.

(1) Result: Father found son to be a competent driver, praised him, went hunting with him, etc., and re-established relationship. Mother found helping to clean up room meant that she cared. Son did most of the work and talked to her about his confusion about girls, which was disturbing to him. Discussions between parents establishing mother's pleasure in work, and father's anger with regard to feeling abandoned, resulted in help at home to get meals started, and better cleaning of home.

7. Follow-up studies reveal task-oriented approach may cause major changes in family's life when there are occasional crises.

8. Some crises are repetitive episodes of severe individual and family decompensation and require long-term continuous intervention. They cannot be dealt with on an episodic basis.

9. Short-term therapy of children and families. Assessment of presenting problems of child and family may indicate that a combined crisis intervention/consultation approach may be helpful.

a) Presenting problems may be chronic but a recent shift in family dynamics - a sibling leaving home, etc. - has altered equilibrium so there is acute discomfort.

b) Major problems presented may focus on normal developmental crisis in an otherwise functioning family.

c) Intercurrent life events, death in family, loss of job, divorce, sibling birth, etc., require period of help to re-establish adaptive strengths in family members.

d) In chronic disorganized families, numerous brief contacts relating to crisis with schools, etc. permit a short period of treatment with minor resolutions to help child or parents function better in one area.

e) In initial assessment, a time limit for the intervention is often set.

10. Therapist's role must be active both in helping family to assess strengths and weaknesses and in helping them to arrive at short-term feasible goals to work on.

a) The question of what one change in family interaction would ease family problems may give some focus to efforts.

b) Analysis with each family member of what tasks other family members could do that would help family to function more smoothly may be helpful.

c) Therapist's activity expresses concern with family and intent to help as well as an authoritative role and expectation that family members will each do their part to help.

(1) Subsequent sessions to determine what did or did not work and why (each family member's version) are important since these issues require clarification and validation.

(2) Use of therapist's authority to help family member who is most oppositional to feel important and to feel that there are expectations of therapist for carrying out of tasks. Need for constant reinforcement and help to get tasks carried out.

(a) Example: A hostile psychotic mother whose school visits caused chaos every time her daughter went to a new school. Mother agreed to call therapist before she went to see principal so they could go together and agreed that principal would be so notified by therapist. Mother made school visits alone, principal called therapist who reminded mother of her task to call him first. After four such unsanctioned visits, the mother called the therapist who came to school with her and helped her through a non-threatening interview to the great relief of mother and principal with some shift in the mother-child relationship.

(3) Assessment of the hurts, fears, angers and longing for closeness and nurturance that are most accessible to surfacing and working on, using recent experiences and recent indications of coping mechanisms within the family.

(4) Resolution of short-term goals requires encouragement and rewards by therapist.

(a) When shift of focus turns from child to family, a similar short-term agreement can be made to work on a pressing present problem which leads to symptomatic behavior in the child.

d) Group therapies most useful in community mental health centers:

(1) Play groups for preschool children.

(a) Especially effective for deprived children who have not had many opportunities to learn to play and explore and have had few toys to use. These children are usually withdrawn or overly aggressive and cannot play by themselves.

(b) Small groups of four to six children with age-appropriate toys, mostly blocks, paints, wheel toys, play dough, music and noisemakers.

(1) Encouraged by adults to learn to use toys

(2) Selection of special toys depending on developmental level and special skills and talents of child

(3) Vocal encouragement by adults to enjoy play and express pleasure

(4) Help to stick with toys which bring pleasure vs. needing to take other child's toys (approval of adults for skills and fun vs. disapproval for encroaching on other children's toys).

(c) When children are able to play with abandon and pleasure with particular toys they can be encouraged to explore other toys. The mastery involved encourages curiosity.

(d) Destructive behavior may be reduced by restraint and disapproval and by providing alternative toys to enjoy.

(e) Gradual lead into parallel play as playing is more spontaneous.

(2) Activity groups for kindergarten through grades 5-6 for children with behavior and learning problems in school related to socializing, i. e., isolation or aggression which results in being left alone.

(a) Purpose of group is to use activities to foster social interaction.

(b) Use of projects, individual and group, to enhance motor skills and developing relationships with adults and children.

(c) Use of restraint to prevent use of tools to injure other children and thus to establish a parenting relationship with an adult whose concern and encouragement toward self-control brings rewarding relationships and increases expression of feelings rather than acting on impulse.

(d) Learning cooperative play.

(e) Learning to recognize and express feelings of anger, hurt, delight, etc. with adults and children.

(f) Use of fantasy group play, storytelling and skits to develop capacity for fantasy expression of both problems and resolutions.

(g) A critical factor is the opportunity to experience with at least two adults and several children a family-like situation with opportunities to experience new aspects of parent and sibling relations.

(h) Use of food before, during and after sessions in various combinations to help decrease oral needs, oral aggression, and need for hoarding.

(i) Beginning of friendships (twosome alliances) as breakthroughs in capacity to experience warm, close feelings.

(j) Reflection of new attitudes toward self and others (social interaction in learning and behavior at school and home).

(3) Early adolescent activity group therapy.

(a) Activity group for adolescents with problems in making friends and in investing self in learning with moderate behavior problems in school and at home.

(b) Focus of group: individual projects, building with wood, jewelry making, ceramics, etc., moving to two-person projects in art, leather work, etc., to group building and mural painting projects.

(c) Moving from group activity projects which require cooperation and developing relationships with adults and other adolescents in talking together.

(1) Adults (at least two leaders in a group) not seen just as parents but as adult authorities from the past who will be arbitrary, capricious, selfish.

(2) Adolescents will attempt to divide adults, ridicule them, render them helpless, to feel superior and repeat ability to defeat parents.

(a) Requires total honesty from adult leaders about feelings evoked and provoked.

(3) Adult's capacity to talk of own feelings and to identify what attitudes, feelings and behaviors of one or more adolescent group members' evoked feelings leads to adolescent efforts to defend themselves by more explicit denial and description of own feelings, ascribing their own feelings to other adolescents, but in the process, the adolescent's own feelings are more clearly defined.

(d) Talking most easily starts with an effort to write a script regarding problems of one group member.

(1) Script is cast and rehearsed with group leaders taking parts and being very dramatic in their portrayal of adolescent, parent, teacher, etc.

(2) Well-rehearsed script is shown to other groups and to parent group.

(3) The process of writing scripts helps state problems and possible solutions to difficult behaviors.

(4) Role playing, spontaneous efforts to solve problems which concern most adolescents in interactions with a variety of adults and peers.

(5) Use of relationships with group leaders and peers to discuss kinds of interactions they enjoy and want.

(6) Efforts at problem-solving in relationships can lead to examining personal goals vs. where their parents are in life.

(7) Practice through role playing of dealing with frustrations of school, job interviews, etc.

(4) Adolescent group therapy for adolescents with behavior disorders, antisocial behavior, drug and alcohol addiction.

(a) Most adolescents with similar behavior problems - adolescent rebellion and efforts at becoming independent and learning to relate to others intimately - will use the group to attack adult authority, sincerity, and honesty.

(1) Such attacks make possible a focus on each adolescent's trouble with some adults like the leader and how they result in problems.

(2) Efforts to involve other adolescents to clarify what is valid and what are excuses and avoidance of reality lead to global discussion of problems and adolescent's feelings of hopelessness in solving them.

(3) Leaders can help with discussions of how people generally learn their behavior which leads to discussion of family problems.

(4) How can adolescents' siblings be helped to stay clear of trouble?

(b) Beginning relationships in group make possible more positive explorations of problems of friendships, couple relationships, and possible solutions.

(1) Parenting issues for adolescents as parents.

(2) What do they want to know about how children develop; how did they and their siblings develop?

(c) In groups with leaders or adolescent participants who are good actors, role playing can be used as part of presenting problems and trying out solutions.

(d) Reduction of symptoms noted outside of group.

(e) Many adolescent groups need to be open-ended and continue while the adolescent practices new roles in society with the support of the group.

(5) Parent group therapy for special groups of parents who have common problems like psychotic children, children with chronic physical illness, retardation, delinquent behavior, adolescent problems, etc.

(a) Effort to share common concerns and experiences with their children.

(b) Examination of what seems to work or not in managing difficult behaviors.

(c) Dilemmas parents find themselves in regarding specific child behaviors:

(1) Anger at repetitive, crazy behavior of child, with guilt and then failure to require decent social behavior.

(2) Guilt when other children accuse parents of favoritism.

(3) Giving in to child's demands, tantrums, suicidal behavior, not taking medication, etc.

(4) Challenges to authority by child.

(5) Disagreement between parents about how to handle a problem; one parent may undermine another.

(d) Problem-solving efforts through discussion, reading of parent information and discussion with local experts.

(e) Group activity and cohesion to obtain better services, education, etc. for children.

(6) Foster parent or group home parents group.

(a) Discussion of common problems with foster children.

(b) Discussion of common feelings elicited by children with specific problems and behavior.

(c) Recognition of being drained by children - what is fair to self.

(d) Discussion and efforts to recognize early signs of giving up on helping a child which usually leads to a crisis and change of home situation; not attending to and dealing with difficult behavior which previously led to intervention.

(e) Discussion of techniques of working with various children using the clues from one's own feelings. Shared learning in problem-solving dealing with one child in one home who is currently at risk.

(7) Parents Anonymous group for abusive and neglectful parents.

(a) Sharing problems about children.
(b) Sharing their own backgrounds and problems in living.
(c) Learning about child development.
(d) Role playing in resolving problem with spouse and with child.

(e) Developing parent hotline and support system.

e) Educative role of children's therapeutic services:

(1) Parent education in parenting,and child development in housing projects.

(2) Education regarding child mental health problems in the community and possible mental health support roles.

(3) Teacher-parent education services on child development learning and mental health.

(4) Primary physician education on child mental health, normative developmental crises and common emotional problems.

(5) Education of primary physicians, minister, etc. regarding counseling with children concerning behavioral problems and chronic and life-threatening disease; similar education on counseling with parents.

f) Collaboration with schools, welfare agencies and courts to facilitate development of treatment and rehabilitation programs with children:

(1) Collaboration with education system to help with recognition of mental health aspects of education.

(a) Teaching and learning problem-solving thinking and methods in elementary grades and throughout the educational process are important for mental health of students vs. feeling of helplessness and impotence in solving any problems from math to social science.

(1) Learn from project research, thinking, and problem-solving processes used in research.

(b) Use of affective learning in curriculum. Identifying feelings in literature, history, etc. and relating them to students', teachers' and parents' feelings to lead to discussions of feelings in human relations.

(c) Using practical learning with seminars like work in day care center and seminar in child development to lead to discussion of parenting, problems noted in children, own experience as child, and kind of parent the adolescent wants to be.

(d) Education efforts tied to learning and thinking about how to solve problems and actual work-study experiences preparing for work and professional roles.

(e) Collaboration with special education regarding treatment needs of very disturbed young children.

(2) Welfare collaboration concerning foster care, unwed mothers, Aid to Dependent Children (ADC) mothers, child abuse and group homes.

(a) Collaboration to actualize mental health potential in welfare responsibilities for children.

(1) Use of emergency group homes rather than large receiving homes to give a personalized, family-like setting to children disturbed by separation from family.

(2) Provide foster and group homes with mental health consultation to deal continually with problems rather than crises, expulsion and transfer of troubled children from one home to another.

(3) Support to unwed mothers on ADC to finish schooling and to learn child care, development and parenting skills with own infant.

(4) ADC mothers with several children to be paid extra to learn new parenting and child development skills with new baby to prevent later disturbance and to alter parenting of older children to increase their mental health.

(5) Child abuse and neglect group foster homes with specially trained foster parents, continuous mental health consultation to several group homes and special mental health services and school services to very disturbed children.

(3) Collaboration with courts to help with developmental assessment of child's needs in custody, divorce, and child abuse and neglect cases.

(a) Help court to make long-term placements in best interest of the child's need to make attachments and durable relationships for optimal development.

(b) Consultation with court to work with families and probationers of first offenders to reduce increasing number of serious offenders.

g) Early intervention and prevention programs in CMHC's:

(1) Use of child development specialists to provide, in collaboration with education or other organizations, early stimulation programs for high-risk youngsters.

(a) Infants with organic deficits - hypermotility, prematurity, sensory deficits, mental retardation and withdrawn infants of depressed mothers - require special developmental assessments and individualized stimulation programs taught to their mothers who should continue clinic program at home.

(2) Parenting programs for infants of high-risk, young unwed mothers require help with nurturing and infant stimulation and feeling rewarded for infant's progress until they feel effective and enjoy parenting.

(3) Early intervention programs by mental health specialists in collaboration with child development specialists.

(a) For preschool children with developmental deviations often noted in sensorimotor disorders or in deprived children with affective relationship problems.

(b) For preschool and young school-age children with hypermotility, withdrawal and beginning psychophysiologic diseases.

(c) Specific remediation programs devised by specialists with attention to developing relationship aspects of remedial program.

(d) Mothers involved in all classes to learn to work with own children, to work with other children with different developmental deviations in order to become more expert at working with a variety of children.

(1) Enhance mental health of disordered children and self-image and feeling of competence of mothers, especially forming a corps of volunteer mothers as early interveners.

(e) Help by mental health specialists to educators and primary physicians and nurses to identify the first signs of psychosocial disturbances followed by joint community mental health center and school intervention and remediation programs.

(1) Early intervention requires awareness of changes in adaptive behavior of children of all ages and

throughout school experience so prompt assessment of problems can occur and treatment, if needed, carried out in collaboration between community mental health center and schools.

REFERENCES

1. Berlin, I. N. A History of Challenges in Child Psychiatry Training. Mental Hygiene 48:558-565, 1964.

2. Berlin, I. N. Working With Children Who Won't Go to School. Children 12:109-112, 1965.

3. Berlin, I. N. Training in Community Psychiatry: Its Relation to Clinical Psychiatry. Comm. Mental Hlth. J. 1: 357-360, 1965.

4. Bindman, A. J. and Klebanoff, L. G. Administrative Problems in Establishing a Community Mental Health Program. Am. J. Orthopsychiatry 30:696-711, 1960.

5. Coleman, J. V. The Contributions of the Psychiatrist to the Social Worker and to the Client. Mental Hygiene 37: 249-258, 1953.

6. Parker, B. The Value of Supervision in Training Psychiatrists for Mental Health Consultation. Mental Hygiene 45:94-100, 1961.

CHAPTER 6

PREVENTION IN COMMUNITY MENTAL HEALTH

Irving N. Berlin, M.D.

1. Definitions of primary, secondary and tertiary prevention

a) Primary prevention is defined as the elimination of a disease disorder before it can occur, by such public health measures as genetic counseling, which might prevent the occurrence of certain kinds of mental retardation. Another measure is providing adequate food and nutrition, protein and vitamins, for a pregnant mother and infant or young child in order to prevent nutritional retardation and other malnutrition-caused developmental problems. The complete prevention of a disease or disorder is still rare in mental health, an example being general paresis due to syphilis, which vanished when the use of penicillin eliminated syphilis as a major disease.

(1) In infants, primary prevention occurs mostly at the prenatal level through efforts at providing adequate protein intake to prevent depletion of brain cells in number and size, and through interference with the pregnancy when certain anomalies or presence of viral disease in mother are discovered. Also during

pregnancy, elimination of drug addiction and alcoholism with their effect on the brain of the infant during the prenatal period is an effective means of primary prevention. There is also some evidence that massive anxiety and psychophysiological disturbance in the pregnant mother may have some effect on the development of the central nervous system of the infant.

(2) In childhood, primary prevention depends upon an awareness of the developmental processes and their facilitation so that parents with problems in nurturing are identified and are helped to learn early parenting skills. They are then able to give their child adequate nurturance in both infancy and childhood, enabling the child to develop normally so his drives toward investigation and curiosity are not disturbed, his capacity for learning is not stunted and there is no interference with the socialization process.

(3) The parents of preschool and school-age children can be helped to anticipate the normal crises of childhood, to understand and deal with these crises as the child leaves the home and goes on to preschool and later to school. These anxieties, which are primarily those of the parents, can be greatly reduced and the psychological difficulties which might otherwise occur can thus be prevented. Later separations in junior high school from a single teacher as parent-surrogate can also be anticipated and worked through for vulnerable children.

(4) In adolescence, primary prevention also occurs by anticipation of the developmental crisis of pubescence with its sexual anxieties and separation and independence problems. A good example of primary prevention in adolescence occurs in colleges, in anticipation of the impact of a large college upon youth from a small town who have previously done very well. Often in college they feel isolated, unable to meet scholastic demands. They become depressed, fail exams, often drop out or attempt suicide.

The college can provide a "buddy" system and dormitory group meetings in an effort to help the new college student become more adapted to college life, to learn how to study, and to deal with the normal problems of the entering student. Such efforts in several schools have greatly reduced the failure rate, the dropout rate (which is almost one-half of entering freshmen in many colleges) and the rate of serious depression and suicide.

(5) Primary prevention in the adult is also centered in the anticipation of the normal adult crises of living - crises stemming from the process of becoming a parent, of having severe illnesses in the family, or of having one or more severe, acute or chronic illnesses oneself as an adult. There are helping professionals who can identify the crisis and anticipate the emotional turmoil which may occur and can help the process of adaptation and coping so that disequilibrium, with its decompensation, does not have to occur as a result of such normative crises of adult life. Other crises such as divorce, moving, death in the family, problems with children throughout the developmental spectrum, and child's leaving home (the empty nest syndrome), reaching 40-50 years of age or retirement may all be causes of severe stress. Through anticipatory guidance, these are areas of potential primary prevention.

(6) The elderly are particularly vulnerable to life changes, retirement often being the first major stress. For this reason, primary prevention of disability in the elderly also depends upon the anticipation of crises that occur when they move from a familiar place to a strange area; when they leave their family, if there is an extended family; and when there is death of a spouse, other relatives, or close friends. In each of these instances, it is possible to prevent severe decompensation if one anticipates the reaction, especially since the reaction may not be an overt one. The effects of each of these severe psychosocial traumas can be

anticipated. It has been clear in some communities that groups of elderly people working together are able to help each other to resolve many of the particular crises they face and, thus, can prevent the severe disorganization and decompensation that may often occur.

b) Primary prevention in relation to secondary prevention. Individual efforts at helping the parent to provide a nurturant environment which is consistent for the child, thus permitting the child to attach to the parent and to form good object relations, are a basis for normal development. Such efforts are just as crucial as primary prevention in babies born normally. The application of these research data to secondary prevention occurs in prematurity. This is one of the crises of infancy in which secondary prevention may be a critical factor in reducing morbidity. There is now sufficient evidence to indicate that involvement of parents in the care of the infant while he is still in the neonatal unit, the stimulation of the infant during his tenure in the unit, and the help of mother working as part of a stimulation program may begin to reduce some of the problems with the infant occasioned by his immature nervous system. Some developmental delays can be successfully reversed. Organic disturbances and mental retardation, when discovered in infancy, may also be dealt with by anticipating the kinds of problems that may occur and developing early programs which will use stimulation of the infant to reduce the severity of the symptoms and to increase the capacity for social relationships and all human interactions.

c) Secondary prevention. By secondary prevention, we mean the very early recognition of a disturbance or disorder and prompt early intervention to prevent serious limitations of the capacity to live and function and to adapt adequately.

(1) In infancy, such secondary prevention occurs by early recognition of the child's temperament, the temperamental fit with the mother, the problems in attachment, and the problems of the mother in nurturing the child which make attachment difficult. In addition, the early recognition of neuropsychological

problems, organic deficits, and maturational developmental lags, which make it difficult for the mother-child couple or parent-child couple to develop an eventually satisfying relationship, permit very early intervention.

Secondary prevention involves helping parents to learn to interact with their child who has developmental problems and to anticipate some of the crises these problems bring about in early childhood. Parents can learn to assist their infant's development by focusing on the particular deficits that each such child presents in infancy. The organic differences in rhythmicity and the temperamental differences can be dealt with in a more positive parent-child relationship when the parents learn how to involve themselves in sensorimotor stimulation which helps organize each child's early development. Later, parents need help to socialize their child by clear, firm and kind discipline. Such firmness about the do's and don'ts become part of living. A child who has reacted to the efforts at stimulation and involvement with the parents by relating more closely to them and making a firmer attachment is then more capable of socialization and has a greater capacity to live with others. These are critical efforts in secondary prevention for children with neurophysiologic and neuropsychologic deficits.

(2) In childhood, secondary prevention occurs on entering and during preschool and elementary school. First, it occurs in the early recognition of the variety of developmental and psychophysiological disturbances. Early diagnosis and early treatment are important in both the medical and the psychological aspects. The child and family need help in accepting the diagnosis and understanding it. They must understand the management problems in each disorder and the problems in living they impose on the child and family. The early discovery of sensorimotor deficits and of learning problems with prompt remediation is critical to the development of the child. Also the

early identification of psychotic disorders or the behavioral precursors to severe neurotic disorders permits early intervention.

(3) In adolescence, secondary prevention occurs primarily through the early recognition of problems in adaptation. Sudden flareups in anger, sudden withdrawal, suicidal threats, and massive withdrawal with implications for psychosis need to be noted and treatment provided. All too frequently depressions of adolescence, if unnoticed, lead to prolonged periods of depression and incapacity to function with failure in school and failure to learn to socialize. Masked depression is noted in drug and alcohol addiction and in some antisocial acting out. It is important to recognize these and begin an intervention program. The early recognition and treatment of these disorders have a long-range effect upon the adaptation of the adolescent and his capacity to function as an adult. A very clear understanding of the developmental process of the adolescent helps one determine the arrests in adolescent development and how the interventions might be planned to be most effective.

(4) Adult, secondary prevention. With adults, early intervention depends upon the early recognition of incipient depression and decompensation as a result of the normal life crises and developmental stresses in persons with previous problems in adaptation. In a nation where the divorce rate is constantly growing and where there is great family mobility, there are additional stresses, as have been indicated by Holmes and Rahe. These stress factors can be used predictively and might form the basis of some early intervention when people are placed under further stress as a result of family illness, disturbances of equilibrium due to problems with children or parents, job loss, and divorce, especially when these are compounded and several occur at the same time. The stress factors may be of such nature that early intervention by mental health personnel, on the recommendation of a physician who recognizes the

at-risk nature of the individuals undergoing such multiple stresses, may be critical. The community mental health center may serve as the resource of the private physician. The early recognition of other life crises such as menopause, issues of retirement, problems which are related to the children's growing up and leaving home, marriage of children and the advent of grandchildren may also be periods of stress for particular individuals. The continuity of care may be possible in some mental health centers when there is no transient population. When the population is known to the center over a period of many years, it may be possible to predict those members of the community who might be more easily stressed as a result of a variety of adverse life conditions. Especially important, besides the stress factors previously mentioned, are unemployment and life events which change one's status in the family or in the community.

(5) Secondary prevention and early intervention for the elderly require the early identification of decompensation. This may involve depression which results from retirement, melancholia reactive to loss of important people, as well as psychotic decompensations due to severe stress such as family loss and sudden unplanned moves to unfamiliar settings. Occasionally depression may be reactive to the slowing down which occurs with age. The effect of retirement and the effect of increased debility and the inability to carry out one's former functions with the same ease may be extremely difficult for some very active and high energy individuals. Early signs of depression and decompensation in the elderly are often signaled by seclusion. "Crank" complaints, or multiple psychosomatic complaints, with unclear psychosomatic symptoms must be looked upon as signs of stress and indications of decompensation that need to be attended to quickly before they become much more serious, debilitating and permanent. Group methods in working with the elderly provide effective early intervention. Often

other group members can detect early signs in their friends who have begun to feel stressed.

d) Tertiary prevention. Tertiary prevention describes the provision of the most effective treatment possible for already existing disorders. The community mental health center should be able to provide the gamut of treatment modalities for all ages ranging from infancy and early childhood stimulation programs to individual psychotherapy in various forms. Tertiary prevention involves family therapy, marital therapy, and group therapy designed for various age groups from latency-aged children, adolescents and adults to the geriatric population. It also includes the assessment of the need for a variety of psychotropic drugs, depending upon the age of the individual and the clarity of the evaluation, as well as the indications for a particular drug for a particular disorder.

(1) In childhood, it is especially important to recognize the fact that the use of stimulant drugs may impede or retard growth and that massive doses of phenothyazines greatly retard the child's capacity to think and to learn. Similarly in adolescents, large doses of phenothyazines may be detrimental to developing integrative behaviors and learning. Again, in the elderly, the psychoactive drugs must be used with some caution, depending upon the physical state of the elderly person. The use of several psychotherapeutic modalities may be necessary to maximize the effectiveness of drugs. Some kinds of group support, as have been found in the day treatment center for adults who have recently been hospitalized for severe decompensations, i.e., psychoses, may make it possible for the elderly to gradually re-enter their family and community and to function more adequately. The use of treatment groups, with discussion about the adaptation of various members and help with jobs and rehabilitation, may make the difference between the successful use of antipsychotic medication and its not being effective in the rehabilitation of the individual patient.

(2) In the adolescent and young adult, the psychosomatic symptoms, particularly psychosomatic illnesses, yield to both a very clear medical regimen and individual or family therapy. This is perhaps most clearly seen in the most severe of psychosomatic disorders, anorexia nervosa. The use of tricyclic medications in depressions has been effective both with adults and with some adolescents, and the use of lithium where there is a history of depressions, especially a history of manic and depressive episodes, has been proven to be effective. A history of manic-depressive illness in past generations makes lithium the drug of choice. Some recent studies show that depressed and psychotic-looking adolescents who have been hospitalized for antisocial acting out with schizophrenic-like symptoms are indeed depressed. Some have a history of manic-depressive illness in the family. A number of these adolescents have done very well on lithium, especially when the blood lithium level is carefully monitored.

2. In community mental health centers, the issues of prevention are hardly dealt with because the primary funding is for direct services. It becomes very clear that there must be some attention to the success of several prevention models in community health centers. There is now sufficient evidence to indicate that an early intervention with infants and young children who have begun to show organic disturbances, either withdrawal or overactivity, and help to their parents to learn to stimulate these infants, has enormous pay-off in terms of development of a mother-child relationship which enables a child to develop normally rather than pathologically, with its subsequent implications for severe disturbance. There is also a good deal of evidence that working with pregnant adolescent girls, and with the same group after their babies are born, does a great deal to help them with the nurturing process so that they can become more adequate mothers and thus feel better about themselves. This, in turn, improves their mental health as well as insures that their children will be adequately nurtured, thus getting them off to a better start with less chance of mental illness. Certainly, in infancy, the issues which have to do with adequate diet, pre- and postnatally, are also critical in terms of prevention of mental retardation and other organic insults to the

newborn. The work of Craviotto and others has indicated that even where there is some organic deficit and retardation, high stimulation programs and stimulation of a concentrated type in the home will greatly alter the capacity of these children to function at a much higher level than their cohorts who are not so stimulated. Attention by the school system to the early warning signs of normative crises in development would help with early intervention and secondary prevention, which is currently ignored. Such efforts could prevent mental illness in many children and adolescents.

a) The mental health center has a critical role to play in integrating its efforts with health care, education and welfare so that the child, adolescent, and adult do not experience fragmented care. Collaboration of agencies is necessary for an integration of the work of professionals on behalf of a child and family or individual. These are also critical issues in terms of the relationship with the mental health center to the courts. The mental health center may be an important resource in helping the court to determine the kind of foster care or residential care, as well as return to the home, which may be in the best interests of the child's development and, therefore, his mental health. The role of the mental health center in helping parents learn to parent and to be more effective, both individually and as spouses, enhances the ability of parents to care for their children, who might otherwise be wards of the court or in foster homes or an institutional setting.

The mental health center's group counseling for parents with problem adolescents, groups for single parents, and for adults with addictions to alcohol or drugs and groups for adults anticipating retirement are all potential prevention activities.

The support of the mental health center to homes for geriatric patients is also critical, since the application of mental health principles in those settings will prevent stress and decompensation for the aged.

Finally, the mental health center's role in consultation with pastors, teachers and health, welfare and court personnel is to recognize disturbances in their clients and counsel them so they can function more effectively in their usual settings.

REFERENCES

1. Berlin, I. N. Preventive Aspects of Mental Health Consultation to Schools. Mental Hygiene 51:34-40, 1967.

2. Eisenberg, L. and Gruenberg, E. M. The Current Status of Secondary Prevention in Child Psychiatry. Am. J. Orthopsychiatry 31:355-367, 1961.

3. Klein, D. C. and Lindemann, E. Preventive Intervention in Individual and Family Crisis Situations. In Prevention of Mental Disorders in Children. G. Caplan (Ed.). New York: Basic Books, 1961, pp. 283-306.

CHAPTER 7

MENTAL HEALTH CONSULTATION

Irving N. Berlin, M. D.

1. Definitions

a) Mental health consultation consists of:

(1) A process of enhancing the professional worker's or administrator's competence in a non-mental health agency or institution by:

(a) Individual meetings with the consultant to discuss disturbing behavior problems in a client or client group.

(b) Group meetings to discuss behavior problems of a client or clients of common concern.

(2) A once-removed method, based on the premise that the worker or administrator has problems with a client group which reflect, at least in part, his or her own personality problems. This method includes:

(a) Discussions which increase an understanding of the sources of the client's problems. These will:

(1) Lead to an exploration of methods of management of the client's problems;

(2) Reduce the worker's or administrator's anxieties and helpless feelings; and

(3) Increase the worker's or administrator's capacity to problem-solve.

(3) Education and imparting of new knowledge which will increase the worker's repertoire of responses to client's behavior.

b) Consultant, consultee and client:

(1) Consultant is the person offering to, selected to or contracted to provide consultation to the personnel of an agency or institution. A consultant may be:

(a) A person with expert knowledge in the mental health field of behavior disorders and manifestation of developmental difficulties or obstacles to the adaptive or optimal functioning of both client group and worker group.

(b) A person with training in the theory and practice of mental health consultation.

(2) Consultee is the recipient of consultation, usually:

(a) The line worker or administrator whose effectiveness and success in a position is obstructed by the troublesome behavior of the client, usually due to personal problems which interfere with his work with the client.

(b) Schoolteachers and principals, probation officers, case workers and supervisors in welfare agencies, etc.

(3) Client is the person or persons who ultimately receive the service of the agency or institution.

(a) Clients may be students, probationers, welfare clients, parishioners, etc.

(b) In instances of administrative consultation, they are the line workers who deliver services to clients and who are responsible to the administrator for their work.

c) General types of consultation:

(1) Technical consultation in which an expert with technical knowledge, not possessed by another group, provides consultation such as:

(a) Surgical consultation to an internist or pediatrician, or psychiatric consultation to a surgeon.

(b) Engineering consultation to an architect on technical problems of the stress capacities of metals, plastics, etc.

(2) Professional consultation in which a more expert professional in an allied profession provides help to a less experienced colleague such as consultation about case management to enhance learning of professional skills. Example: consultation by a psychiatrist to social workers in a social service agency.

(3) Mental health consultation which enhances the problem-solving capacities of a consultee by reducing internal obstacles to working with difficult clients.

2. Purposes of mental health consultation

a) Communication of mental health principles to a variety of health, education, welfare and justice organizations in the community and to religious and service organizations. For example:

(1) Child-serving agencies in a community may be helped to consider a developmental mental health orientation as part of their function.

(2) The community may be better served by organizations which have a mental health orientation in their work.

b) Consultation extends the range of effectiveness of mental health workers:

(1) It aids agency workers responsible for client groups to work more effectively with client groups.

(2) It aids in solving the special problems of clients of consultees.

c) Groups served:

(1) Welfare workers;
(2) Probation workers, both juvenile and adult;
(3) Public health personnel;
(4) Teachers;
(5) Members of administrative staff in a school, agency or system;
(6) Pastors of congregations; and
(7) Service organizations (Scouts, Campfire Girls, Big Brothers, etc.)

d) General orientation of mental health consultation:

(1) Consultees learn to deal with their clients more effectively by understanding the origin of their clients' problems.

(2) Consultees learn to select ways of working with their clients and to practice those ways.

(3) Through practice and analysis of efforts, consultees become more skillful in helping their clients to function better.

(4) Many difficult clients who otherwise would be seen in a mental health system can be dealt with in a variety of other front-line systems.

3. Brief history of mental health consultation

a) Coleman, in the early 1950's, first described his work with a welfare department and a private social service agency:

(1) He demonstrated that previous methods of acting primarily as an expert who advised consultee how to work with a client more effectively, based on psychodynamic principles, seemed ineffective since they did not reduce the number of clients with similar problems brought to consultation.

(2) He pointed to the need to concentrate on the anxieties generated by the client and to try to reduce these.

(3) He developed some methods to help the frontline workers (consultees) utilize their increased awareness of clients' problems and reduce their own anxieties in order to work more effectively with difficult clients.

b) Coleman described some possible agency-specific problems:

(1) In the welfare department, the problem of the dependency of the clients on the workers resulted in anger when their needs were not met, since dependency meant loss of freedom to act in one's own best interest.

(2) Subsequent work by Caplan, Berlin, Susselman, Bigson and others also indicated that there might be some specific issues in a probation department, namely, authoritarian vs. authoritative role of probation officers:

(a) The need to defend oneself against hostile and frightening feelings generated by aggressive, antisocial clientele, both adults and children.

(3) Caplan described the problems of authoritative use of power in a public health department:

(a) The enforcement of public health laws and regulations may result in difficulties for those who see themselves in a helping role and not in the role of an authority.

(4) Caplan, Berlin, Parker, and others noted that problems in the education system may relate primarily to the anxiety created when learning and behavior problems interfere with teaching and learning. Thus, teachers may be thwarted in their educational- and growth- and development-promoting role.

4. Development of methods

a) Gerald Caplan, in the early 1950's, described his experiences in consultation and his development of a method of consultation devoted to a brief crisis-type intervention:

(1) Essentially, he described a method of handling problems presented by the consultee in dealing with a client's behavior.

(a) The once-removed method emphasizes focusing on the client who presents these problems to the consultee - not directly on the consultee's problems.

(2) Caplan delineated the process of theme interference, that is, the individual neurotic obstacles within each consultee which make it difficult for him to carry out his particular task with a client population:

(a) A focus on a client with problems similar to a consultee's specific conflicts permits a once-removed, less threatening discussion of consultee's problems.

b) Beulah Parker, in the late 1950's, described a similar process in nursery schools and in a public health department:

(1) She delineated a much more educative role for the consultant:

(a) The imparting of knowledge which was previously not part of the consultee's experience.

(b) The presentation of increased options open to the consultee.

(c) Increasing an awareness of how problems are generated in clients.

(d) Reducing self-blame for the consultee because of inability to help the client.

(e) Indicating that the consultee's frustrations with a client are shared by others in a similar position.

c) Susselman described his work with a probation department:

(1) Probation officers tend to bend laws which make their job more difficult and to ignore the judge's explicit rulings.

(2) Illegal acting-out of their clients is encouraged when workers behave illegally with regard to the judicial decision imposed on the client.

d) Berlin, in his early papers, 1955-1956, described essentially a similar kind of mental health consultation method oriented toward a continued process rather than a brief consultation. Later, he described a process using a scientific experimental design.

(1) All process consultations take at least several months and consist of six general phases:

(a) Contract development;
(b) Relationship development (promotion of collaboration);
(c) Data gathering regarding consultee and client behaviors;
(d) Intervention generating and testing;
(e) Consolidation; and
(f) Termination

e) Caplan later delineated several varieties of mental health consultation and made explicit his methods of consultation which have been widely adopted.

5. Types of mental health consultation. Caplan described three general types of mental health consultation:

a) Consultee-centered consultation. This type of consultation includes both individuals and groups:

(1) It provides help to the consultee on specific problems, and it depends on the mutual agreement that the consultee does, in fact, need help in these areas.

(2) Caplan specified that part of the job of the consultant was education, broadening the knowledge of the consultee and dealing with theme or neurotic interferences, which make it difficult for the consultee to carry out his job. The consultee, through his own efforts, may be about to resolve the problem, but requires brief help in consolidation.

b) Client-centered consultation. Individual and group discussion is about a client of the consultee who presents problems:

(1) Discussion of the client provides opportunities to enhance the capacity of the consultee to work more effectively. This permits reduction of theme interference and obstacles to work with the client.

c) Program-centered consultation. The mental health consultant is asked to help with the mental health aspects of a program in a particular agency.

(1) The issues are delineated by the administration, sometimes with the help of committees of lineworkers.

(2) There is usually a specified length of time given to the mental health consultant.

(3) He presents to the administration or the group of representatives of the agency a plan for altering the program to enhance its mental health components.

6. Mental health consultation process

a) The process of mental health consultation has good validation through intensive and extensive trials:

(1) It is an effort by the mental health consultant to help a worker from another profession to work more effectively with a difficult client group.

b) The method involves:

(1) Diagnostic appraisal of the conflicts in each consultee and between a consultee and a client that cause the work problem.

(2) Development of a dynamic understanding of the consultee's underlying anxieties and the form in which they are presented to the consultant; understanding of the dynamics and capacities of the client.

(3) Assessment of the integrative capacities of the consultee; assessment of the ego strengths and capacities of the client.

(4) Use of various approaches to reduce anxieties and form a working relationship by the consultant's interaction (collaboration) which indicate:

(a) His understanding and sympathy with the consultee's problem;

(b) His acceptance or range of feeling with respect to client's behavior or demands placed on administrator as consultee; and

(c) His acceptance of conflicts engendered in the consultee by the behavior of the clients.

(5) Discussion of how similar problems have, or may be, handled by others. The consultee is then able to try some of these methods to experience whether or not they can be effective in dealing with the problems of the client.

(6) Review one's interactions with the client and change methods of work with client as required.

c) Group consultation: a similar process:

(1) The group usually selects a client problem common to most members of the group.

(2) The individual who volunteers to present this problem frequently speaks for the entire group.

(3) In this process various group members, through identification, learn how they can work with their own clients.

(a) They participate in the consultant's efforts to help the consultee with the problems of his client.

(b) They attempt to use the variety of methods suggested to alter a client's behavior.

(c) As they learn to be more effective, their personal obstacles (theme interference) to understanding and dealing with specific disturbing client behavior are reduced.

7. <u>General phases in mental health consultation</u>

a) The development of a consultation contract with the agency requesting consultation. This includes:

(1) Clarifying the needs, purposes and pressures which initiated the consultation request.

(2) Clarifying the terms under which the mental health consultant will work with the consultee.

(3) Ensuring that consultees have been consulted and want consultation and have agreed to meet with the consultant at mutually convenient times.

(4) Clarifying the purposes of consultation as seen by the consultant:

(a) To work on particular problems of consultees concerning clients or groups of clients.

b) Despite the contract,

(1) Often there is no recall of the initial agreements; and

(2) The consultation contract must be worked out by the consultant simultaneously with the administration and the consultee or consultee group as a part of a process of engagement in consultation.

c) In initiating consultation, the primary goal is the establishment of a relationship with the consultee or consultee group.

d) The mid-phase of consultation occurs when the consultee:

(1) Has agreed to participate in the consultation process.

(2) Is comfortable with the consultant.

(3) Is able to suggest and to carry out the recommendations which are agreed on by both the consultant and consultee in an attempt to alter the behavior of the client.

(4) Is able to accurately observe and report back the effects of interventions agreed on in consultation.

(5) Is able to alter intervention to ensure maximal effectiveness.

e) The end phase of consultation occurs when:

(1) The consultee is able to work effectively with several clients with similar difficulties.

(2) The consultant and consultee agree that objectives of consultation have been met.

(3) The consultant and administrators agree that consultation objectives have been met.

8. <u>The scientific or experimental models of mental health consultation: stages in the model</u>

a) The first stage consists of those initial efforts at the development of a <u>collaborative</u> relationship:

(1) To begin mutual efforts to understand the client.

(2) To use these efforts to reduce self-blame and anxiety with respect to client and awe and fear with respect to consultant.

(3) To begin the process of data collection:

(a) Consultees usually resist data collection because of the time and effort it requires.

(b) They must be involved in it in order to gather the pertinent facts which permit:

(1) Hypothesis generation; and
(2) Problem-solving.

(4) Collaboration occurs through the consultant's efforts to demonstrate human understanding and empathy with the consultee and the problems presented.

b) The second phase occurs after most of the data have been collected:

(1) The consultant and consultee review the data carefully.

(2) They begin to assess what factors in the past through the present seem to have determined the client's problems.

(3) They determine what current issues in the client's life lead to or increase behavioral difficulties.

(4) A behavioral data basis is established for critical review of the client's behavior:

(a) During the day with specific time frames like:

(1) Upon entering class;
(2) During academic work;
(3) Before recess;
(4) After lunch; and
(5) At end of the day.

(b) Interactional or social data base:

(1) Problems occur with whom and when; and
(2) Reactions to authority vs. lack of firmness and authoritative behavior of adults occur.

(5) In this process, the consultee becomes the primary observer and reporter of data.

c) The third phase is hypothesis generation:

(1) Both consultant and consultee consider data from the past and the current data which has been collected by the consultee from daily observations.

(2) They generate hypotheses about what makes the difficult behavior occur at particular times with certain people in terms of the developmental behavioral data obtained from home and school.

(3) Hypotheses are then constructed about what is necessary for reversing the process.

(4) From several possible intervention hypotheses one is chosen to be experimentally tried.

d) Testing the hypothesis:

(1) The data from the intervention are examined in an effort to test the hypothesis that has been generated.

(2) After the analysis of a number of trials, alteration of the hypothesis occurs to fit current observed behaviors.

(3) Ultimately a hypothesis is developed to fit both data on causes of behavior disturbances and effective intervention.

e) A method of dealing with the disturbing behavior is finally worked out:

(1) The consultee learns how to deal effectively with that behavior. Similar interventions can be applied to clients with similar problems.

f) Final phase of consultation using the experimental model occurs when the consultee is able to:

(1) Apply the method of data collection;
(2) Analyze the data;
(3) Generate a hypothesis;
(4) Test the hypothesis;
(5) Refine the hypothesis;
(6) Work out an effective intervention; and
(7) At this point, work with client is ended.

9. <u>Obstacles to consultation in the consultant/consultee relationship</u>:

a) Introductory phase:

(1) Consultee's unreal expectations of consultant as obstacles to collaboration:

(a) Belief in consultant's omnipotence, a desire for easy answers.

(b) Fear of being exposed as inadequate which may be fostered by consultant's glib psychodynamic formulations of the client's problems.

(c) Belief in consultant's ability to influence administration on consultee's behalf.

(d) Demand for instant answers to behavior problems of client and the consultant's effort to satisfy these demands so that a process of consultation is delayed.

(e) Anger and disappointment when consultant tries to maintain a consultative collaboration and develop a process to enhance the consultee's functioning; demands placed on consultee to work.

(f) In group consultation: the expectation is that the consultant will be expert in learning or educational processes other than only behavior.

(1) Refusal to accept limited expertise as applying to understanding origins, causes and interventions for behavior problems.

(2) Education expertise is in the group of educators and available to them.

(2) Consultant's unreal expectations of the consultee:

(a) Countertransference feelings towards adults in authority, teachers, etc. as yet unresolved, especially with administrators.

(1) Sees administrators with childlike awe and fear.

(b) Expectation of easy collaboration.

(1) There is a need quickly to reduce anxiety, and the fear of consultee about being analyzed.

(2) Expectation of easy collaboration often results in a sense of irritation and personal failure because the consultant is not immediately effective.

(c) Belief in one's own omnipotence with disappointment that suggested solutions do not work or were already tried.

(d) Lack of experience and conviction about a process of consultation with phases in which a problem-solving collaboration must be established; belief that a brief crisis encounter consultation will not usually do more than help resolve a single crisis.

(e) Narcissistic hurt when in early phases consultee's problems are not easily resolved; consultant withdraws his affect and energy and the relationship deteriorates.

b) Middle phase or problem-solving collaboration:

(1) Consultee's problems:

(a) A major problem in this phase is the consultee's growing dependence on the overly sympathetic consultant whose help has been effective and who has catered to the helplessness of the consultee and not required and facilitated a real collaboration.

(b) Consultee's feeling of success and effectiveness is based on a single success.

(1) Desire to do it alone, be independent.

(2) Fear of dependency thus ending consultation before learning how to deal with the class of problems that are most difficult.

(c) Consultee's use of consultant against authority by misconstruing his comments and involving consultant as authority in a fight with the administration.

(2) Consultant's problems in mid-phase:

(a) Failure to recognize Hawthorne effect of early success and ending consultation before it is consolidated and consultee has demonstrated capacity for using what was learned in a number of ways with different students.

(b) Consultant's failure to observe that consultee reports success but appears anxious and tense. This may be due to:

(1) Internal anxieties about new learning and needing to be helped after initial success; or

(2) External pressures from co-workers or administrators hostile to the consultation process.

(c) Consultant's lack of experience in psychotherapy and consultation. A sense of the time required for a change in behavior to become operative and part of the consultee's armamentarium.

(d) Countertransference problems with very authoritarian or very dependent consultees.

(1) Tendency to become hostile or feel defeated.

(2) Inability to maintain an on-going consultative relationship.

(3) Special anxiety with rough, hostile, angry consultees who abuse children.

c) End phase of consultation:

(1) Problems of consultee and consultant are similar, a reluctance to let go of a comfortable and productive collaboration and to go on by oneself and to help others more in need.

10. New developments

a) Greater use of program consultation to special programs in agencies with large mental health components:

(1) Example: Special education consultation, students with many severe psychosocial problems.

b) Shifts in technical consultation:

(1) Example: Pediatric liaison consultation is not only for help with diagnosis or treatment recommendation of pediatric client, but also a request for help in dealing with ward personnel, specialty medical professionals regarding altering their mental health attitudes and capacities to work with sick children.

c) Consultant as educator and consultant with mental health professional and paraprofessionals learning to work with community groups.

REFERENCES

1. Altrocchi, J., Spielberger, C. and Eisdorfer, C. Mental Health Consultation with Groups. *Comm. Mental Hlth. J.* 1:127-134, 1965.

2. Berlin, I. N. Transference and Countertransference in Community Psychiatry. *Arch. Gen. Psychiatr.* 15:165-172, 1966.

3. Berlin, I. N. and Szurek, S. A. (Eds.). *Learning and Its Disorders*, Vol. I. The Langley Porter Child Psychiatry Series. Palo Alto: Science and Behavior Books, 1966.

4. Berlin, I. N. Consultation and Special Education. In I. Philips (Ed.). *Prevention and Treatment of Mental Retardation.* New York: Basic Books, 1966, pp. 279-293.

5. Berlin, I. N. Mental Health Consultation for School Social Workers: A Conceptual Model. *Comm. Mental Hlth. J.* 5:280-288, 1969.

6. Berlin, I.N. Some Lessons Learned in 25 Years of Mental Health Consultation to Schools. In S.C. Plog and P.I. Ahmed (Eds.). Principles and Techniques of Mental Health Consultation. New York: Plenum, 1977, pp.23-48.

7. Bernard, V.N. Psychiatric Consultation in the Social Agency. Child Welfare 33:3-8, 1954.

8. Bindman, A.J. Mental Health Consultation: Theory and Practice. J. Consult. Psychol. 23:473-482, 1959.

9. Caplan, G. Types of Mental Health Consultation. Am. J. Orthopsychiatry 33:470-481, 1963.

10. Coleman, J.R. Psychiatric Consultation in Casework Agencies. Am. J. Orthopsychiatry 7:533-539, 1947.

11. Gibb, J.R. The Role of the Consultant. J. Social Issues 15:1-4, 1959.

12. Haylett, C.H. and Rapoport, L. Mental Health Consultation. In. L. Bellak (Ed.) Handbook of Community Psychiatry. New York: Grune & Stratton, 1963.

13. Hollister, W.G. Some Administrative Aspects of Consultation. Am. J. Orthopsychiatry 32:224-225, 1962.

14. Kevin, D. Use of the Group Method in Consultation. In L. Rapoport (Ed.) Consultation in Social Work Practice. New York: Nat'l. Assoc. Soc. Workers, 1963, pp. 69-84.

15. Lippitt, G.L. Operational Climate and Individual Growth: The Consultative Process at Work. Personnel Administration 23, 1960

16. Maddux, J.F. Psychiatric Consultation in a Public Welfare Agency. Am. J. Orthopsychiatry 20:754-764, 1950.

17. Newman, R.G., Redl, F. and Kitchener, H.L. Technical Assistance in a Public School System. Washington, D.C.: Washington School of Psychiatry, 1962.

18. Rosenfeld, J.M. and Caplan, G. Techniques of Staff Consultation in an Immigrant Children's Organization in Israel. Am. J. Orthopsychiatry 24:42-62, 1954.

CHAPTER 8

MENTAL HEALTH EDUCATION AND PUBLIC INFORMATION

Richard M. Yarvis, M.D., M.P.H.

1. Efforts at education which seek to disseminate information about mental health should have as their aim the enhanced understanding of mental health concepts by a broad public audience. If such efforts are successful they will:

   a) Facilitate increased knowledge about measures which if applied can prevent the occurrence of mental illness (i.e., the introduction of suitable child-rearing practices and appropriate, rapid attention to individuals who are exposed to stress).

   b) Facilitate increased knowledge about what early signs and symptoms constitute mental illness. Such knowledge if applied can lead to the early identification and treatment of mental illness (i.e., self-recognition of impairment or the recognition of mental illness by family, doctor, clergyman, spouse, or parent when the impaired individual attributes his or her difficulties to other causes).

   c) Facilitate increased knowledge of what treatment services are available. Information about how and where to obtain suitable treatment services if applied can lead to treatment of the mentally ill (i.e., the most well-motivated person cannot attend to treatment needs if he or she has no awareness of what help is available or where it is located).

d) Inculcate attitudes about mental illness, the mentally ill and their treatment across the broadest public spectrum so that impaired individuals are willing to utilize available treatment facilities (i.e., a recognition that mental illness is treatable and a perception of mental health professionals as benign helping resources).

e) Inculcate attitudes about mental illness and its treatment among family doctors, clergymen, teachers and others to whom the mentally ill commonly turn first for help so that these "gatekeepers" are willing to refer impaired persons to available treatment facilities (i.e., the willingness of a clergyman or a family doctor to refer parishioners or patients to mental health treatment settings).

f) Inculcate attitudes about mental illness and the mentally ill so that mentally ill persons enjoy greater tolerance in their communities and within their own families (i.e., a greater willingness to accept mentally ill persons in the community and to treat them there instead of isolating them in massive state hospitals where they can remain out of sight and out of mind).

2. In order to accomplish the above, the following available data must be examined:

a) Current knowledge about attitudes toward mental illness and mental health treatment.

b) Factors which have led persons *not* to seek help for emotional problems.

c) Primary gatekeepers to whom mentally ill persons turn first and those factors which influence the referral practices of such gatekeepers.

d) Factors which facilitate or which thwart informational enhancement or attitudinal change in the public.

e) Results from experimental efforts to influence attitudes about mental illness or mental health treatment.

3. What do we know about the public's knowledge about mental illness and its treatment?

a) The best data available to answer this question are to be found in a study conducted by Nunnally.[1] Three random samples of adults were surveyed in each of three different communities. Randomly selected psychologists and psychiatrists were also surveyed.

b) By asking the community and expert samples identical knowledge questions, "what the public thinks" could be correlated with "what the experts think."

c) Nunnally's salient findings include:

(1) High correlations between public informational beliefs and those of experts in most areas. While gaps in public knowledge were apparent, there was little evidence of public misinformation.

(2) Public information and expert opinion were most divergent in the areas of how to maintain or to re-establish mental "equilibrium." The public tended to support the utility of willpower, denial and the "power of positive thinking" more than the experts did.

(3) The public's informational reservoir was not highly structured nor was it highly crystallized. There was a high level of uncertainty about information, and opinions were readily changeable.

(4) Several subgroups within the public sample were significantly more misinformed. These included persons with less than high school educations and persons 50 years old or older.

(5) The experts themselves generally agreed with respect to two items; however, significant disagreement was demonstrated. These items were:

(a) The best methods of psychotherapy; and

(b) The primary etiologic causes of mental disorder.

d) In general, confirmation of these findings comes from another similar study by Elinson and his group.[2] Elinson obtained similar data from a random sample of 2118 adults living in New York City.

e) The implications of these findings for mental health education programs are:

(1) That correcting misinformation in the public mind will not be the primary task of mental health education efforts.

(2) That filling in gaps in information will be necessary and will be possible since current information is not highly crystallized and is apparently open to augmentation and change.

(3) That certain groups within the population, especially the less educated and the older age groups do have significant levels of misinformation which should be corrected. Since the elderly are a high risk group for mental health problems, this kind of re-education effort will be especially important.

(4) That a potential for public confusion regarding preferable treatment techniques exists because the experts disagree. This fact must be carefully considered in the design of all mental health education projects.

4. What do we know about public attitudes toward the mentally ill and toward treatment for mental illness?

a) Both of the above-cited studies examine the public's attitudes toward mental health. In both studies, attitudes are generally negative.

b) Nunnally found in the population he surveyed that:

(1) The mentally ill were generally regarded with distrust and were frequently viewed as worthless, dangerous, unpredictable and untrustworthy; and

(2) Such negative attitudes characterized all socio-economic and demographic groupings with only a small difference between more and less well educated persons. This is in contrast to the more striking differences in knowledge between these two groups.

c) Elinson and co-workers concur with and illustrate Nunnally's findings with the data presented below:

(1) Note how responses become progressively more negative as the closeness of the association with the mentally ill person increases (Table 1).

TABLE 1

If you find out that a person has been a patient in a mental hospital, would you be willing:

	% Yes	% Qualified	% No
To work next to him	72.9	13.8	12.3
To have him as your boss	44.3	15.7	37.7
To have him live next door	69.3	12.1	17.6
To share an apartment with him	23.2	17.5	57.4
To take such a person into your home for $150/mo.	11.1	13.4	73.2

(2) Note also how clearly the widespread fear of dangerousness and the sense of distrust can be demonstrated (Table 2).

TABLE 2

	% Agree	% Disagree	% Don't Know
It is unfair to the women and children of a community to mix mental patients among them.	43.6	49.1	7.3
Most women who have gone to mental health clinics could be trusted as baby-sitters	28.1	55.3	16.7

(3) Finally note the sense of shame that pervaded many respondents with respect to mental illness within their own families (Table 3).

TABLE 3

	% Yes	% Qualified	% No
When mental illness happens to a family it is wise to keep it a secret as far as possible.	32.3	65.2	2.4

d) The implications of these findings for mental health education programs are:

(1) That attitude change will be a primary task of any mental health education project.

(2) That fear and distrust permeate the public's view of the mentally ill and that these issues should constitute an important focus of education projects.

(3) That families are apt to hide their own mental health problems and that in some instances this undoubtedly reduces the likelihood that help will be sought. To increase the frequency with which persons seek help, such attitudes must be combated.

e) The data presented above were collected ten or more years ago. There is, however, little to suggest that such attitudes are no longer prevalent in wide segments of any population, as can readily be seen by reading any local newspaper.

5. The view of the public toward mental health professionals and toward mental health treatment facilities will certainly influence their willingness to utilize such professionals and facilities. How does the public feel about the providers of mental health treatment?

a) Once again the best available data come from the same studies by Nunnally and Elinson.

b) Both studies note a moderately positive public attitude toward mental health professionals and treatment in general.

c) Psychiatrists appear to rank fairly high in public esteem according to both studies but below that of other physicians.

d) Nunnally finds few distinctions in the public mind between psychiatrists and other mental health professionals such as psychologists and social workers. Elinson, on the other hand, finds that psychiatrists enjoy a higher level of prestige and are thought to be more qualified to treat the more severe forms of mental disorder.

e) When psychiatrists are compared with other medical specialists in Elinson's study, they do as well or better with respect to their interest in patients and their knowledgeability. However, they are related strikingly worse with respect to their success in helping patients (Table 4).

TABLE 4

	% More	% Less	% Same
Interest in welfare of patients	33.1	4.1	56.8
Knowledge of mental and emotional conditions	74.5	2.7	18.2
Success in helping patients	23.5	15.1	48.6

f) Neither study assessed the public's view of the quality of care in community mental health settings but Elinson did examine some aspects of quality in other settings.

(1) Ratings of the chances that a patient will get better if treated in a state hospital were fairly optimistic (Table 5).

TABLE 5

Chance of Getting Better	% Responding
Good to Excellent	42.6
Fair	34.1
Poor to Very Poor	17.1
Don't Know	6.2

(2) When state hospital care is compared with care in a general hospital, however, it fares less well (Table 6).

TABLE 6

	% Responding	
Quality of Care	State Hospital	General Hospital
Good to Excellent	39.3	51.9
Fair	32.3	34.4
Poor to Very Poor	18.3	8.5

g) The implications of these findings for mental health education projects are:

(1) That the public's view of mental health professionals is basically positive and need not be stressed in education projects.

(2) That much needs to be done to counteract the public's lack of faith in the success of mental health treatment. The lack of agreement among experts on what constitutes appropriate treatment undoubtedly contributes to this and more consistency in this should be sought.

(3) That even ten years ago the public had more faith in the general hospital (community care) than in state hospital care. Hence, community mental health programs have an important positive opinion base on which to expand their notions of community care.

6. Attitudes consistent with utilizing treatment facilities are certainly important but, without an awareness of where and how to find facilities, no treatment can take place. What then do we know about the public's awareness of existing mental health treatment facilities?

a) Turning first to the already cited study by Elinson we find that his respondents cite ignorance of available sources of help as a common reason why persons do not go for help. In fact, 24% of his respondents cited this as a reason.

b) To test this, Elinson asked respondents to identify by name some mental health facility that serves New York City residents. The results which are presented below bear out the notion that <u>the public is not well informed about available treatment resources.</u>

<u>Informed about available treatment resources</u>

38%: could not correctly name a general hospital with psychiatry beds in New York City
57%: could not correctly name any state hospital that serves New York City residents
73%: could not correctly name any mental health clinic in New York City

c) Another study carried out in 1957 by Gurin and his co-workers[3] on a national sample of 2460 randomly selected adults also contributes data to this issue. Gurin found that <u>20% of those who did not seek out treatment for problems failed to do so because they lacked knowledge about means.</u>

d) In a more recent study Heineman and co-workers[4] assessed public awareness of local community mental health facilities. They found that:

(1) Only 15% of respondents were aware of the existence or location of the local community mental health center; and
(2) Awareness by residents living within 1/2 mile of six satellite clinics ranged from 10-62% with a mean of 32%.

e) Elinson's data also offer us insight into where people look for information about what services are available. Mental health education efforts must disseminate information about available facilities and services to and through those sources which people consult most frequently (Table 7).

TABLE 7

From whom would you get the name and address of a source of help?	% of responding
Physician	37
Telephone directory	16
Church or clergyman	13
Friend	9
Hospital or clinic	6
Mental health facility	4
Family member	3
Social agency	3
Lawyer, judge, court	2
Medical society	2
Professional directory	1
School or teacher	1
Mental health professional	1
Mental health society	1

Obviously family physicians, the telephone directory and clergymen are prime foci through which to disseminate information.

f) The implications of these findings for mental health education projects seem eminently clear. Public awareness of available facilities is sparse and is undoubtedly an important contributor to nonutilization. All community mental health centers must consider the need to mount active public information programs which saturate their communities with information about available treatment services.

7. Mental health education programs would be well served by some knowledge of the kind of persons who are most and least likely to seek out help for mental health problems. Armed with such data public education projects can be selectively directed at unlikely help seekers.

a) Our best national data come from Gurin and coworkers whose study has already been cited.

b) Gurin found that the likelihood of help-seeking:

(1) Decreases as the education level achieved drops;
(2) Decreases in adults as age increases;
(3) Is greater in females than males; and
(4) Is greatest in separated and divorced persons and lowest in widows.

c) The implications of these data are clear enough. Education efforts should be specially aimed at older persons, males, persons with less education and widows. The notion that such groups might be less likely to need help is not borne out by other available data (see chapter on Epidemiology).

d) Several recent studies have challenged a pervasive notion that minority groups are less motivated to seek out help for emotional problems than are other groups. These studies[5, 6] suggest instead that the quality of services and the reception that such groups sometimes receive account for decreased utilization rates where such occur.

8. Another issue that is worth exploring relates to reasons why persons fail to seek out help in spite of some recognition

that it is needed. Again, we turn to the work of the Elinson and Gurin groups to illustrate this issue.

a) Gurin and co-workers asked the 220 persons in his sample of 2460 who thought they needed help but who did not seek it out to cite one or more reasons for not doing so. A distillate of responses are recorded on the right-hand side of Table 8.

TABLE 8

Reasons that respondents believe will prevent others from seeking help (Elinson, et al.).	% citing	% citing	Reasons that respondents gave for not seeking out needed help for themselves (Gurin, et al.).
Shame or embarrassment	45	14	Shame or stigma
No faith in or need to rely on self-help	11	7	Would not help
		25	Emphasis on self-help
Cannot afford it	30	4	Cannot afford it
Shyness or temporizing	42	Nothing comparable cited	
Fears about treatment	39	Nothing comparable cited	
Lack of insight	28	6	It will go away by itself

b) Elinson and co-workers asked their entire sample of 2118 to offer opinions as to what kinds of things would commonly prevent persons from seeking out needed help. A distillate of their responses are recorded on the left-hand side of Table 8.

c) Note that the categories used in the two studies are not identical in all cases. Note also that Gurin was asking people about their own actual experience while Elinson was asking people to speculate about what might motivate others. Hence each study has approached the same question from a somewhat different vantage point.

d) Comparing the studies, note that neither cost nor shame is as potent a dissuader as respondents in Elinson's study speculated that it would be and that the emphasis on self-help is more important than they thought it would be.

e) The data suggest that mental health education efforts might do well to focus on the appropriateness of seeking assistance and of not having to feel that only self-help is acceptable.

9. Mental health education efforts ought to be focused on those professionals to whom the public actually turns for help. The right kind of educational efforts so directed should aid such helpers to be maximally effective in assisting the mentally ill. To whom does the public turn for help?

a) Data to answer this question are provided, once again, by Elinson and Gurin. They are presented in Table 9 and represent the actual experience of the respondents.

TABLE 9

Helping source (Gurin - National Sample)	%	%	Helping source (Elinson-N. Y. City Sample)
Clergyman	42	4	Clergyman
Family physician	29	20	Physician
Psychiatrist or psychologist (private and public settings)	18	66	Psychiatrist or psychologist (private and public settings
Other practitioners or social agencies	10	7	Social worker
Lawyer	6	3	Lawyer
Marriage counselor	3	7	Counselor

b) Note the dramatic differences between the use of psychiatrists and psychologists and the use of clergymen in the two studies. We must assume until other data are available that Gurin's study is more reflective of national trends but that Elinson's data may be of more use to programs located in large urban settings.

c) The family physician clearly deserves more of the time and attention of mental health education efforts than he now gets.

d) At least from Gurin's data, clergymen also warrant intensive exposure to mental health education efforts.

10. Mental health education programs must focus special attention on so-called gatekeepers, agencies, professionals, and others in the community to whom persons in need of help turn first and who in turn either provide help directly or refer such persons to some other source of help.

a) The gatekeeper about whom the most is known is the family physician but the practices and attitudes of other gatekeepers will be examined as well.

b) Nunnally's study, already cited previously, is one of those which looked at the relationship of general practitioners to mental illness and to the mental health treatment system. Summarized, his findings indicate that:

(1) General practitioners do definitely serve as gatekeepers between the public and psychiatrists.

(2) Such practitioners treat a sizeable projection of mentally ill patients themselves.

(3) They tend to have generally correct information about mental illness but do tend to have the same negative attitudes toward the mentally ill that the general public has.

(4) They have a generally favorable opinion toward mental health professionals, methods and institutions.

c) In a series of four reports[7, 8, 9, 10] drawn from studies of patients enrolled in a prepaid health care program, Fink, Goldensohn, Shapiro and Daily investigated how primary care physicians deal with mental health problems and what impact the establishment of a community mental health program has on such practices. Summarized, the findings from these studies reveal:

(1) That prior to the establishment of the community mental health program patients referred to psychiatrists tended:

(a) To have chronic rather than acute problems;

(b) To have conditions that the physician regarded as "important"; and

(c) To have conditions that interfered significantly with life functions.

(2) That subsequent to the establishment of the community mental health program with its active encouragement of referrals:

(a) The utilization rate of mental health treatment services increased by more than 50%;

(b) More acute and more "less seriously" impaired patients were referred for care;

(c) Patients with a wider range of problems were referred for treatment; and

(d) The primary care physicians used a wider range of treatment techniques (especially drugs) on patients that they themselves treated, indicating they had learned about these techniques from the mental health center staff.

(3) This group's findings also suggest that almost half of the patients seen by mental health experts got there primarily because of the primary care physician's influence and not as a consequence of self-referral.

(4) Their evidence also suggests that patients referred by physicians are frequently "new" patients who have never been seen before and who would not have tended to be referred by any other source:

(a) These patients fail to recognize the need for treatment;

(b) They tend to come from population groups who traditionally avoid psychiatric care; and

(c) They would come to the attention of a psychiatrist much later in the course of their illness.

d) A study by Dohrenwend, Bernard and Kolb,[11] while quite old, sheds interesting light on the attitudes of four different groups of community leaders with respect to mental illness. This study should be replicated to check on the validity of its findings but is interesting enough to bear mention here.

(1) Leaders were selected from four different areas: education, politics-law, religion and economics-business. Using a set of case histories and related questions, these groups were assessed for:

(a) The tendency to discern the person in the case history as mentally ill;

(b) The tendency to label the illness described as serious; and

(c) The tendency to recommend treatment by mental health professionals for each case example.

(2) The findings for each group are summarized in Table 10.

TABLE 10

Leadership group	Tendency to identify person in case history as mentally ill	Tendency to label the illness as serious	Tendency to recommend psychiatric treatment
Educational	high	high	high
Political-legal	high	low	high
Religious	low	high	low
Economic-Business	low	low	low

e) What is the significance of all these studies to the design and implementation of mental health education programs?

(1) Primary care physicians must be a prime target for mental health education efforts because:

(a) Such activity on the part of a community mental health program greatly influences the number of referrals such physicians make to psychiatrists;

(b) Such referrals are made earlier and for patients with less severe illnesses who ostensibly are at more correctable stages of illness;

(c) The primary care physicians reached and referred patients not usually referred or self-referred to mental health settings; and

(d) The primary care physician had a wider array of treatment techniques at his own disposal as a result of such education efforts and apparently used them.

(2) Primary care physicians apparently start out with attitudes toward the mentally ill which are as negative as those of the general public. Since they are clearly important gatekeepers and a prime resource for many in need of help, more positive attitudes on their part toward the mentally ill are critical. Mental health education programs should seek to influence such negative attitudes.

(3) The data on leaders from various groups lead to several conclusions:

(a) Educational leaders tended to relate most sensitively toward mental illness. This suggests a fertile climate in the schools for screening programs and early interventions. Moreover, it suggests that mental health education efforts directed at patients are likely to have the support of the educational system and perhaps should be conducted under the auspices of that system.

(b) The political-legal group was also fairly sensitive to mental health issues. More thought should be given to mobilizing the prestige of such leaders behind mental health education programs.

(c) The clergy were fairly insensitive to mental health issues. This warrants intensive corrective educational programs because the clergy are important gatekeepers and are frequently sought out by persons in need of help.

(d) The least sensitive group were the economic-business leaders. This group also requires corrective educational programs because they are frequently in positions of power with respect to funding for mental health programs and because rehabilitative efforts require reintegration of the mentally ill into the community; the latter certainly includes the occupational area. Businessmen who harbor very negative attitudes toward the mentally ill are unlikely to cooperate in such rehabilitative efforts by hiring patients and expatients. Rehabiltative and preventive programs which attempt to counter the increasing stresses and pressures on workers of modern industrial life are unlikely to garner the support of businessmen who harbor such negative attitudes.

11. Finally, we must look at some examples of mental health education programs which have been tried and at some additional data which may be of help in designing future programs.

a) One of the earliest and best known of such projects was that devised by Cumming and Cumming[12].

(1) Two small communities in central Canada were selected for scrutiny. One was exposed

to a six-month barrage of news stories, radio programs, films, specials, PTA programs, library displays and so on.

(2) Scales were selected to measure tolerance for the mentally ill and social responsibility for them and measurements made before and after the education campaign in the exposed and control communities.

(3) No demonstrable impact of the education campaign could be observed in the exposed community to differentiate it from the control community.

(4) The Cumming and Cumming study, while well known and widely quoted, has simply left us with many unanswered questions.

b) In another study of ways to influence attitudes about mental illness, McGinnies, Lana and Smith[13] exposed adults to films on mental health.

(1) Groups of women were exposed to one, two or three films on mental health. Some groups were further exposed to post-film discussions and others not.

(2) A mental health opinion inventory of 47 items was used to measure attitude change pre- and post-exposure.

(3) This study determined that exposure to only one film had little impact but exposure to the entire set of three films produced significant improvement on inventory scores. Discussion groups did not have any discernible impact.

c) Balser, Brown and Brown[14] focused another mental health education project on school administrators and teachers:

(1) They exposed these professionals to a series of lectures on mental health by a psychiatrist, each followed by a discussion period.

(2) Both the exposed group and a control group were matched for sex, age and other factors.

Pre- and post-measurements of knowledge and personal adjustment were made.

(3) No increments in knowledge were noted in either exposed or control group. Both groups showed significant increments in the adjustment measures which suggests that participation in the study influenced the results.

d) As can be seen from the above examples, the impact of mental health education programs has been mixed. Such programs have frequently raised more issues than they have resolved.

e) Nunnally, whose study has already been cited, also described experiments in which he examined alternative methods of presenting mental health information and for influencing attitudes. His findings are summarized:

(1) With respect to attitude change, Nunnally found that:

(a) Attitude change (after some communication process) does not correlate well with personal characteristics such as age, sex and intelligence;

(b) Communication efforts can transmit mental health information effectively but will not so easily affect attitudes; and

(c) Favorable mental health attitudes are more likely to occur when people think they know something about mental illness than when they do not, regardless of whether the beliefs they hold are right or not.

(2) With respect to capturing an audience and fostering attitudinal change, Nunnally found that:

(a) Mental health topics are moderately interesting but less so than severe physical problems (heart, cancer, stroke, etc.).

(b) People want to know such things as what causes mental illness, how to recognize it and what can be done about it;

(c) The personal aspects rather than the broad social aspects are of interest;

(d) The presentation of information which tends to allay anxiety and at the same time offers information about causes, early signs and treatment is most likely to gain and keep an audience;

(e) High anxiety messages tend to promote unfavorable attitudes about mental health;

(f) Where high anxiety is evoked in a message, the presentation of "solutions" at the same time results in more favorable attitudes;

(g) The more certainty with which a message is offered, the more impact it will have;

(h) Misinformation should not be simply negated but actively replaced with new information.

(3) Nunnally demonstrated with his data that brief messages properly constructed with non-threatening and informative content can have a lasting impact on mental health attitudes.

12. As can be seen from this chapter, much work remains to be done in the area of mental health education. There are many unanswered questions about preferable target groups, and about the preferable content and techniques to be employed. The material offered above provides many clues as to the direction in which such future work should proceed.

REFERENCES

1. Nunnally, J. Popular Conceptions of Mental Health. New York: Holt, Rinehart and Winston, Inc., 1961.

2. Elinson, J., Padilla, E. and Perkins, M. Public Image of Mental Health Services. New York: Mental Health Materials Center, Inc., 1967.

3. Gurin, G., Veroff, J. and Feld, S. Americans View Their Mental Health. New York: Basic Books, 1960.

4. Heinemann, S., Perlmutter, F. and Yudin, L. The Community Mental Health Center and Community Awareness. Comm. Mental Hlth. J. 10:221-227, 1974.

5. Ring, S. and Schein, L. Attitudes Toward Mental Illness and the Use of Caretakers in a Black Community. Am.J. Orthopsychiatry 40:710-716, 1970.

6. Karno, M. and Edgerton, R. Perception of Mental Illness in a Mexican-American Community. Arch. Gen. Psychiatr. 20:233-238, 1969.

7. Fink, R., Goldensohn, S., Shapiro, S. and Daily, E. Treatment of Patients Designated by Family Doctors as Having Emotional Problems. Am. J. Public Hlth. 57:1550-1564, 1967.

8. Fink, R., Shapiro, S., Goldensohn, S. and Daily, E. The Filter Down Process to Psychotherapy in a Group Practice Medical Care Program. Am. J. Public Hlth. 59: 245-260, 1969.

9. Fink, R., Shapiro, S., Goldensohn, S. and Daily, E. Changes in Family Doctor's Services for Emotional Disorders after the Addition of Psychiatric Treatment to a Prepaid Group Practice. Medical Care VII: 209-224, 1969.

10. Fink, R., Shapiro, S. and Goldensohn, S. Family Physician Referrals for Psychiatric Consultation and Patient Initiative in Seeking Care. Soc. Sci. and Med. 4:273-291, 1970.

11. Dohrenwend, B., Bernard, V. and Kolb, L. The Orientations of Leaders in an Urban Area Toward Problems of Mental Illness. Am. J. Psychiatr. 118:683-691, 1962.

12. Cumming, E. and Cumming, J. Closed Ranks: An Experiment in Mental Health Education. Cambridge, Mass.: Harvard University Press, 1957.

13. McGinnies, E., Lana, R. and Smith, C. The Effects of Sound Films on Opinions about Mental Illness in Community Discussion Groups. J. Applied Psychol. 42:40-46, 1958.

14. Balser, B., Brown, F. and Laski, L. Further Report on Experimental Evaluation of Mental Hygiene Techniques in School and Community. Am. J. Psychiatr. 112:199-205, 1955.

CHAPTER 9

MENTAL HEALTH MANPOWER

Donald G. Langsley, M.D.

1. When the National Institute of Mental Health (NIMH) was established, it was given the triple responsibilities of service to the mentally disordered, research on basic and applied programs for mental health, and the education of mental health professionals and paraprofessionals. The subsequent development of community mental health programs and the specialized personnel who staff them has had a profound effect on both the locus and types of services being provided to the mentally disordered. Mental health programs depend upon people (staff) rather than on machines or special physical facilities. Therefore, the quality of care in a CMHC will vary with the skill, knowledge and sensitivity of those who provide the services.

2. Numbers of mental health manpower

   a) Psychiatrists were recognized to be in short supply during World War II, when Congress and government leaders viewed with dismay the large number of military personnel being rejected or relieved from active duty because of mental illness. The training of more psychiatrists became a national priority, evidenced by federal budgetary appropriations for expanding such training programs. With this effort, the number of psychiatrists has increased from an estimated 5,000 at the close of World Was II to between 25,000 and 30,000 today. Of those 25,000 (members of the American Psychiatric Association), approximately 17,000 are in actual practice; the others being involved in administration, research, teaching, and other activities.

b) Other mental health professions include the clinical psychologists, clinical (sometimes called psychiatric) social workers, and the psychiatric/mental health nurses. Along with psychiatrists, these are called the four "core" mental health professions. Numbers of practitioners within each group over the past three decades are shown in Table 1.

TABLE 1

	Psychiatrists[a]	Psychologists[b]	Social Workers[c]	Registered Nurses
1950	7,100	7,300	20,000	(not available)
1960	14,100	18,200	26,200	504,000
1970	23,200	30,800	49,600	722,000
1980	28,000	45,000	72,000	1,000,000

[a] Estimates from the American Medical Association
[b] Membership of the American Psychological Association
[c] Membership of the National Association of Social Workers

These figures represent personnel who are licensed and/or registered in their respective fields, and do not necessarily reflect the number of individuals working directly with mental health patients. Still, the numbers clearly indicate how rapidly each of the four "core" mental health professions has expanded during the past 30 years, while our society's demand for their services has increased at an even greater rate.

c) Community mental health centers were designed to use multi-disciplinary teams, including the four core disciplines, plus others as described below. One of the most startling changes in CMHC's since 1970 has been in the "mix", or ratio of representation among the four disciplines. The number of full-time equivalent psychiatric staff per CMHC has dropped from 6.8 in 1970 to 4.3 in 1976, and at this moment, more than 50% of CMHC's have fewer than 2.3 psychiatrists. During that same six-year period, there was a concomitant doubling of psychologists (from 4.9 to 8.6 per center); and a 35% increase in social workers (from 9.7 to 12.8). This growing gap between medical and non-medical CMHC staff ratios has alarmed mental health professionals and paraprofessionals alike, many of whom originally proposed or supported the CMHC concept. Their concern is that CMHC's with severely diluted physician representation will not be able to deliver the full range and quality of services they were designed to provide and upon which communities have come to depend.

d) Changes in the original CMHC model have evolved since the 1969 publication, Action for Mental Health, and the 1963 Kennedy message to the nation. In part these changes have been adaptations to fundamental shifts in leadership. Psychiatrists are no longer the directors of such centers; more frequently one sees professional managers (individuals with education and training in hospital or health care administration) and/or social workers becoming the administrative directors of a CMHC. Another leadership change is reflected in the move toward consumer control, with CMHC governance boards composed of community members. This is a major departure from the original CMHC model, wherein centers were sponsored by existing health care agencies (such as community hospitals) whose own boards governed the CMHC. The implications of citizen groups forming non-profit corporations to operate community-based (not hospital-based) CMHC programs are yet to be fully understood and assessed.

3. Categories and roles of mental health professionals and other personnel

a) Psychiatrists are MD's who have had four to five years of training following medical school. The physician-psychiatrist is presumed to have special skills in:

(1) Comprehensive evaluation, including the organic causes of mental illness and the psychiatric complications of organic disease;
(2) The management of psychiatric emergencies;
(3) The competent use of psychoactive medications;
(4) The use of other physical treatments for mental illness;
(5) The treatment of mental illness in a hospital setting; and
(6) The role of consultant and educator to other physicians.

Psychiatrists are again becoming a shortage specialty due to decreasing numbers of American medical college graduates entering the field, and to the recent curtailment of foreign medical graduates being permitted to enter the USA for residency training. An especially negative consequence of this situation has been the erosion of the psychiatrist's role in CMHC's. Some centers have reported that the function of their staff psychiatrists has been reduced to merely signing prescriptions. Furthermore, the psychiatrists in many CMHC's are employed on a part-time basis, and thus are not as well integrated into the mental health team as they should be in order to assure a reasonable quality of overall care. As with other mental health professions, there are distressingly few minority practitioners, totally inadequate numbers of child psychiatrists and geropsychiatrists, and a geographic distribution problem which often leaves rural areas completely deprived of psychiatric care resources. Depite the need to attract more psychiatrists to CMHC's, there has been a drop in the proportion of psychiatric trainees in CMHC's from 29% to 14% of the total. In view of the fact that psychiatrists are absolutely necessary to treat those with psychoses and other major mental disorders, and because they are needed to consult with the primary care physicians who treat 55% of those with a clear diagnosis of mental illness, the shortages work to the disadvantage of patients and the whole system. It would be desirable to increase the amount of training of psychiatrists carried on in such centers to acquaint more young psychiatrists with the possible careers available to them.

b) Clinical psychologists are individuals with degrees at the Ph. D. or Psy. D. level (with a few M. A. -level exceptions) who have special training and skill in:

(1) The assessment of psychological functions;
(2) The application of psychological principles to the resolution of mental disorder;
(3) Consultation in the broad area of mental health; and
(4) Research design and implementation

The past three decades have seen a more dramatic expansion in the number of psychologists than of any other mental health profession. The American Psychological Association has experienced a rise in membership from 7,300 in 1950 to over 42,000 in 1976. Including those with master's level degrees, there are as many as 70,000 psychologists in the USA; however, there are many other disciplines in psychology besides clinical (e.g., experimental, industrial, etc.) represented in that number. Fifty-seven percent of the psychologists are engaged in part-time or full-time private practice. The geographic distribution of psychologists closely follows that of psychiatrists. Psychologists have been moving into mental health service programs in large numbers for the past 20 years, and are active in therapy, administration, mental health consultation and research. An observed trend among psychologists has been the move toward behavioral therapies (in clinical practice), and toward mental health program planning and evaluation (in administration). Psychologists are trained in university programs (generally leading to a Ph. D. degree); and in recent years, certain professional schools of psychology have been developed to offer the Psy. D. degree. The American Board of Professional Psychology oversees professional certification, but a number of states have their own boards of licensure for psychologists.

c) Social work provides a variety of social and human services including:

(1) Professional casework generally identified as psychotherapy and/or counseling;
(2) Services to encourage or sustain optimal social functioning;

(3) A special knowledge of family and community functioning; and
(4) A special knowledge of community resources directed toward social services

The National Association of Social Workers lists about 70,000 members (increased from 20,000 in 1955), but there are many others with the B.A. level training who function in social work settings. In 1976, approximately 31,000 social workers were employed in public mental health facilities according to NIMH statistics, representing a ten-fold increase in four years. Social work has a higher proportion of minority practitioners than psychiatry or psychology; and interestingly, the proportion of men has been steadily increasing. Although social workers use the same basic skills as other mental health professionals, their field shows more emphasis on group work and community process. More social workers are found in administrative areas, and they are now the largest professional group to be found among directors of CMHC's. The Council on Social Work accredits the social work educational programs. Individuals with the ACSW designation have completed supervised experience beyond the basic professional training and have passed additional examinations.

d) Mental health nursing (also called psychiatric nursing) is the standard designation for that group of nurses who have specialized in the mental health area. They have generally achieved the M.A. level in education and are skilled in:

(1) Working with patients in hospital settings and hospital milieu therapy where nursing relationship skills are required in addition to usual nursing skills related to dispensing medications;

(2) Generic evaluation and treatment in outpatient settings; and

(3) Administrative and leadership responsibilities in working with other mental health personnel in hospital and clinic settings

There are approximately 1,000,000 nurses in the USA, of whom approximately 180,000 belong to the

American Nurses Association. Some 29,000 of those are categorized as psychiatric/mental health nurses.

e) Pastoral counselors and chaplains are clergymen who work in mental health programs and/or perform special work in counseling the mentally disordered. Some are employed as chaplains in mental hospitals and others are employed by CMHC's, while still others work as parish ministers and spend much of their time counseling parishioners or congregants. There are special training programs in pastoral counseling and national organizations for accreditation and certification. Pastoral counselors in CMHC's often provide professional supervision to parish ministers involved with counseling, and they also coordinate the referral of patients from churches to CMHC's and other mental health settings.

f) Occupational therapists use activity experiences as therapy to treat patients with functional disabilities. They are also involved in evaluation and treatment planning. Such therapists receive undergraduate and graduate training, and may be registered as OTR's after completing various requirements which include supervised clinical experience. Their activities are designed to rehabilitate the patients as opposed to simply keeping them busy.

g) Recreational therapists are involved in the rehabilitation of patients through prescribed recreational programs. They may use specialized adjunctive techniques such as art, music or dance therapy. Such individuals are usually trained at the M.A. level and work in institutional programs. Some are found in CMHC's, often in partial hospitalization programs. In the USA, there are approximately 1,000 members in each therapeutic category: art therapy, dance therapy and music therapy.

h) Vocational counselors are involved in assessment, counseling, retraining and placement of mentally and physically disabled persons. Since vocational rehabilitation is important to the chronic mental patient, increasing numbers of such therapists are found in CMHC's.

i) Special education teachers receive graduate special training to work with the physically and mentally disabled. An important group with which they work are the mentally retarded. Hospitals and mental health centers involved in the treatment and rehabilitation of children are primary employers of special education teachers.

j) Paraprofessionals are a diverse group of mental health workers whose formal training is at the high school graduate or Associate Arts degree level, although some have baccalaureate educations. Paraprofessional programs have been developed in response to local needs of mental health and human services agencies, and as part of the "New Career" initiatives. Such workers (many of whom are regularly recruited from minority groups) tend to be classified by functional job titles rather than by occupation or education. They work in all types of settings, from CMHC's to mental hospitals to aftercare programs. They provide a variety of services to the mentally ill, drug abusers and alcoholics, most of which focus on social support, social activities and reality-oriented counseling. The origins for this new mental health specialty field can be traced to the psychiatric aides, orderlies and technicians who have long been the backbone of mental hospital staffs. There is no national credentialing program for the paraprofessionals, but efforts are underway to devise job descriptions based on competencies. Because many paraprofessionals view their work as a career springboard, opportunities for obtaining mobility within their classifications, more clearly defined job descriptions, and more education in order to qualify for the professional classifications are issues being addressed within their organization.

k) Indigenous healers are prestigious individuals from minority cultures who are sought out in times of illness and stress. They include Indian Medicine Men, Curanderos of the Mexican-American cultures, and the "granny ladies" of rural black cultures.

l) Self-help group workers are persons who have themselves been victims of mental disorder or similar problems, and who encourage patients to organize activities and programs to help themselves. Examples are Alcoholics Anonymous and a variety of drug abuse programs. They may work independently or in cooperation with mental health professionals.

m) Volunteers are individuals who offer their time and skills in activities which range from custodial work to counseling and activity therapies. Many serve as part of an organized body (sometimes formed by the local mental health association), while others offer their services as individuals. In both cases, they are an important part of the mental health system.

4. Issues for mental health manpower

a) What types and numbers are needed? As previously mentioned, the diminishing numbers and functional activities of psychiatrists in CMHC's are especially critical problems to be addressed. Unfortunately, there are others, such as the problem with part-time psychiatrists who are more likely to identify themselves with their private practice than with the center. Also, many of the psychiatrists in CMHC's are individuals from other countries whose difficulties in understanding the language and cultures of the CMHC patients are all too apparent. If CMHC's are to take seriously the responsibility of treating all of the mentally ill in their particular catchment area (including the seriously ill who are too frequently transferred to state hospitals), then their staffs must have appropriate leadership and effective clinical guidance. Psychiatrists must provide the clinical direction in centers offering treatment for a broad range of psychological and somatic problems, and they must take more responsibility for the treatment of the most seriously ill. They must also be involved in the triage and diagnosis of difficult cases, as well as the ongoing education and consultation/supervision of other medical and nonmedical staff. Regrettably, national standards for CMHC staffing have not yet been developed. One of the criteria for evaluating quality care in CMHC's will be linked to minimum staff requirements, and this will include the delineation of numbers and activities for each profession to be represented.

b) What roles for paraprofessionals and volunteers? There is abundant evidence upholding the effectiveness of paraprofessionals and volunteers in providing supportive services to mentally ill persons. It is not true, as some have suggested, that these individuals are being used in place of professionals to lower costs. Definitions of roles according to levels and areas of competence are needed, however, if these persons are to be of help to patients and if they are to avoid disorganization and competition within disciplines of the team. As mentioned before, job definitions, credentialing, financing of training and illuminating new career pathways for paraprofessionals are key issues for these groups and for the whole CMHC movement.

c) Relationships to primary care physicians. Studies done for the President's Commission on Mental Health have shown that 58% of the mentally disordered are seen in the general health sector, that an additional 22% are seen by human services personnel or receive no treatment at all, and that only 20% of the "mental patients" are actually seen and treated by mental health professionals. Under these circumstances, CMHC's and their mental health personnel (especially psychiatrists) must learn to work closely with primary care physicians in the general health sector. Systems must be developed for providing early consultation on complex psychosomatic cases, and for teaching primary care physicians about the treatment of those mental conditions which can be managed successfully by them.

d) Social services or health models? Some have suggested that the proper place for the CMHC movement is within social services rather than health. Actually, the CMHC's relate closely to the social and human services, but they have always been part of the health system. Indeed, funding for mental health programs does not come from welfare, but from health. The complex relationships between psychosocial and biological factors in mental and physical illness have always indicated that mental health is not separable from general health. The move toward aligning CMHC's with social services instead of health has generally come from those who are against medical leadership per se, and from those who oppose biological or somatic treatments of mental disorder. Often, these are also the groups who would have us believe that mental illness is due entirely to social problems such as poverty, racism, delinquency, etc.

e) Geographic maldistribution. The shortage of psychiatrists and psychologists in rural areas and in some inner cities is widely known and the development of appropriate models to treat such population areas is an important item on the national agenda. To draw more mental health professionals into the rural areas, training programs have been allowing students to conduct part of their education in those areas, in hopes that familiarity with their people and the environment will encourage them to return after graduation. Closer communication with more urban CMHC's has been suggested as an approach to the inner city's unmet needs. Traveling mental health teams have been helpful in attending immediate problems, but more long-range solutions to distribution problems must be found.

f) Foreign medical graduates were once relied upon heavily as a resource for offsetting psychiatric manpower shortages. By 1975, 39% of all psychiatric residents were foreign graduates. In various years, over 50% of the staffs of some mental hospitals have been FMG's. But it was found that differences in language and culture (which are so vital to effective communication) pose problems that are more difficult to overcome in mental health than in physical health. The recent Health Manpower Legislation has markedly diminished the number of FMG's that may be trained in the USA, and even those training opportunities are limited to individuals who will return to their own country. The vacancies which will be created in service systems once manned by FMG's are new problems yet to be faced.

g) Shortage of services for select populations. A number of population segments are exceedingly short of manpower for mental health services. There are approximately 2, 800 child psychiatrists in the USA, whereas at least 12, 000 are needed by the most conservative estimates. Shortages in mental health manpower for the elderly are also critical. Fully 25% of the population will be over 65 by the year 2000; yet only a handful of psychiatrists have special training in the psychiatric problems of the aged. The minorities are significantly under-represented on CMHC professional staffs; and we do not have enough effective programs for increasing minority representation and for "sensitizing" the existing staffs to the special needs of minority populations. Prisons are "holding compounds" for thousands of mentally ill, yet these institutions are seriously lacking in adequately trained psychiatric personnel and effective mental health programs.

h) Public-private practice. Though many mental health professionals begin their careers by working in organized settings (such as CMHC's), they are frequently drawn away by the financial rewards and professional autonomy of private practice. This turns out to be one of the major sources of tension between the various mental health professions. Groups, as long as they remain organized as such, seem to find ways of working together in the team setting; but when one or more of the team splinters off into private practice, a degree of competitiveness is generated. It is this internecine competition which has been troublesome. Private practice is also a problem because the isolated mental health professional in private practice cannot offer patients the variety of treatments which may be required to meet his particular needs. For the non-physician, there is often a tendency to avoid somatic therapy since it means referring the patient to another professional. For the physician in solo practice, there must be certain limits on the number of seriously ill patients he can treat. The drift towards private practice also drains the public sector (CMHC's and state mental hospitals) of needed personnel.

i) Quality control and competency assurance. The public is entitled to some assurance that those professionals who are treating them are competent. Yet professional competence, especially in the mental health field, is sometimes difficult to measure. Several issues raised over the past few years include:

(1) What degree of individual competence is required of those practicing psychiatry?

(2) What degree of individual competence is required of those providing other mental health services?

(3) How is that competence measured?

(4) How do such factors as training, experience and personal qualities relate to competence?

(5) How do we ensure that practitioners keep current about and avail themselves of new therapeutic techniques developed in their fields, as well as skill mastery programs and opportunities for advancing their knowledge base?

There are no easy answers to any of these problems, but they must be faced and solved. Continued neglect and avoidance are not alternatives. If the mental health professions do not meet these challenges squarely and implement necessary reforms and changes, the opportunity to do so will pass from our hands into those of political figures and special interest groups. National currents in favor of strict quality control and accountability in all health systems are rising; and the laws and regulations produced under such circumstances have traditionally ignored patient needs, professional opinion, and in some cases common sense, in favor of cost containment. The only alternative, therefore, is swift cooperative efforts among mental health leaders, efforts to solve these problems and to protect the interests of those most dependent upon us: our patients.

REFERENCES

1. Koran, L. Psychiatric Manpower Rations: A Beguiling Numbers Game. Arch. Gen. Psychiatry 36:1409-1415, 1979.

2. Langsley, D. G. and Robinowitz, C. B. Psychiatric Manpower: An Overview. Hosp. and Community Psychiatry 30:749-755, 1979.

3. Liptzin, B. The Psychiatrist Shortage: What's the Right Number? Arch. Gen. Psychiatry 36:1416-1419, 1979.

4. Pardes, H. Future Needs for Psychiatrists and Other Mental Health Personnel. Arch. Gen. Psychiatry 36: 1401-1408, 1979.

5. President's Commission on Mental Health. Report to the President from the President's Commission on Mental Health. Washington, D. C.: Superintendent of Documents, 1978, Vol. I, pp. 35-41, and Vol. II, pp. 411-496.

CHAPTER 10

HIGH RISK POPULATIONS

Richard M. Yarvis, M.D., M.P.H.

1. A high risk population is one that can be identified by some common characteristic and in which:

   a) A higher prevalence of mental illness can be demonstrated than can be demonstrated in the general population; and

   b) A higher than average risk for the development of mental illness pervails.

2. Being at high risk does not automatically insure that mental illness will occur. In fact, only a minority of those who are at high risk will actually become ill.

3. Why then is it useful to focus on high risk populations? Such a focus provides the best possible opportunity for a mental health center to:

   a) Design preventive programs which are specific to the needs of those groups _most likely_ to develop mental illness. The impact of such programs will be to reduce the likelihood of illness occurring.

b) Design programs for early intervention (e.g., crisis intervention) which can limit the longevity of illness that does occur and minimize the occurrence of sequelae from those illnesses.

4. Three different research approaches have attempted to delineate and explore the issues around high risk populations:

   a) One approach has focused on the relationship between stressful life events and the occurrence of mental illness.

   b) A second approach has examined data from large epidemiological studies of mental illness in order to discover subgroups within the larger population that are afflicted with mental illness at selectively higher rates.

   c) A third approach has focused on particular mentally ill patient groups or on groups exposed to a particular stress (e.g., the loss of a parent during childhood) to look for relationships between the stress and subsequent patient status.

5. Before we turn to each of these approaches in more detail, we must define two critical concepts which are important for an understanding of high risk status:

   a) Vulnerability is a term which distinguishes individuals who are more likely to become mentally ill if exposed to some stressful life event from other individuals who are less likely to become ill. A number of factors may contribute to increased vulnerability in any particular individual.

      (1) Genogenic factors: the gene pool that a person inherits undoubtedly contributes to his or her risk of mental illness. One or two mentally ill parents would appear to increase vulnerability.

      (2) Psychogenic factors: the impact of parents, other significant persons and the immediate developmental environment on the developing child contribute ego strengths or defects. These will augment or weaken coping capacity and hence aid or hamper the individual's capacity to master life stresses.

(3) Sociogenic factors: the impact of more global and less immediate social, cultural and economic features of a person's environment will enhance or retard his or her capacity to cope with life stresses. Economic, cultural and social supports, where present, serve as important coping adjuncts; where absent, they appear to increase vulnerability.

b) Exposure is a term which refers to the phenomenon wherein a particular stress is inflicted upon an individual. When that individual is less vulnerable, his or her capacity to cope with the stress will be relatively great. When the individual is more vulnerable, exposure is more likely to lead to an inability to cope with the stress and that, in turn, to mental illness. Two types of exposure can be differentiated:

(1) Exposure to the ubiquitous stresses of life, the expectable stresses. These include the birth of a sibling, the beginning of school, marriage, childbirth, the loss of elderly loved ones, retirement and so on. These ubiquitous stresses offer a mixture of desirable and undesirable happenings. They are linked to normal development and maturation.

(2) Exposure to unexpected, out-of-the-ordinary stressful events. These might include events like sudden death or injury, assault, being robbed, the death of a child and so on.

6. We will introduce a variety of high risk groups that either have increased vulnerability or who have been exposed to some stressful situation. We will examine the evidence for their high risk status as provided by one of the three research approaches cited previously. We will show how knowledge of their high risk status is useful to a community mental health program.

7. As was noted previously, one approach to the study of high risk status utilizes the findings of studies which have sought to define the relationships between life change and stress on the one hand and mental illness on the other. Such studies have used one or another variant of the life event checklist to uncover either retrospectively

or prospectively a relationship between social, economic, environmental and interpersonal events and the symptoms and signs of mental disorder. Such studies have evolved out of earlier studies which sought to relate stress and physical disease.

a) Documentation of the relationship between stressful life events and the onset of mental illness has come from a variety of clinically oriented patient-related studies, only some of which shall be mentioned here.

(1) Brown and Birley[1, 2] compared the occurrence of stressful events in a group of schizophrenic patients at various intervals prior to the onset of an acute psychotic episode. They found that such events had occurred at a significantly higher frequency only in the three-week interval immediately preceding the acute psychotic episode. Events were measured which were independent of patient control and hence could not be attributed to some early effect of the psychotic state. Measurements of life events in a normal control population at other points in time showed no significant difference with the schizophrenic group except in the interval already noted above. Brown and Birley's data show a clear association between an increase in stressful life events and the onset of a psychotic episode.

(2) Smith[3] looked at admissions to a mental health center and noted a high correlation with the occurrence of two particular life events: divorce or separation and the onset of alcoholism in a family member.

(3) Paykel,[4] studying the same phenomena, has noted the following:

(a) That stressful life events do occur at a significantly greater rate before the onset of psychiatric disorders than at other times;

(b) That this is true for events which are independent of the persons and hence could not simply be early manifestations of the illness;

(c) That such events are most frequently associated with suicide attempts, then depression and then schizophrenia;

(d) That in neurotic patients a linear relationship can be demonstrated between the amount of stress and the severity of the disorder;

(e) That the shortest temporal relationship between stress and onset of the disorder is found with suicide attempts; and

(f) That stressful life events lead to disorder in a minority of persons.

b) Community surveys which examine general populations rather than patient populations have also demonstrated an association between stressful life events and psychiatric disorder.

(1) Dohrenwend[5] studied 124 heads of family that made up a representative sample of residents from the Washington Heights area of New York City. Using the Langner screening scale to identify psychological disorder and a life events checklist to determine the frequency of life events, she demonstrated a strong association between the frequency of such events and psychological impairment. Again the association is demonstrable even when only events not controllable by the person are examined.

(2) Myers and co-workers[6] in New Haven have used the same methodology, albeit slightly different instruments, to examine these relationships in 720 New Haven adults. These investigators also show an association between the number of life events and the prevalence of emotional disorder. Myers made two sets of measurements in the same population at two-year intervals and replicated the earlier findings two years later.

c) The finding that an association exists between the occurrence of stressful events and the onset of mental disorders has led to much discussion as to whether it is the event itself or some quality of it that matters. Two major points of view have evolved. Neither has had the last word yet.

(1) One hypothesis argues that change from a steady state and the requirement of some kind of life adjustment account for the relationship. This hypothesis suggests that neither the psychological meaning nor the desirability or undesirability of the event is critical.

(a) The original proponents of this hypothesis are Holmes and Rahe[7]. One of their studies[8] carried out with 2458 U.S. and 1056 Norwegian seamen demonstrates the association between life events and illness. Each event was rated and given a readjustment score and it was these scores that correlated best with psychological impairment.

(b) The study by Dohrenwend in Washington Heights cited previously reports data which support the hypothesis of Holmes and Rahe.

(2) The other major hypothesis suggests that the desirability or undesirability of an event rather than change and the need for readjustment that it requires is responsible for the association with mental disorder. According to this hypothesis the psychological meaning of an event is important.

(a) The work of Myers and his group and that of Paykel cited previously both support this hypothesis. Both have found undesirable events to be the only ones associated with mental disorder.

(b) Gersten[9] in a study which looked at children and young adults came to the same conclusion.

(c) Vinokur and Selzer[10] working with data obtained from two groups of male drivers could find only correlations between undesirable events and a number of instruments which measure psychological impairment.

8. A second approach to the study of high risk status utilizes the findings of some mental illness epidemiological studies. Since some epidemiological studies have looked not only at impairment rates in the general population but within specific subgroups within the population as well (age specific, socio-economic specific and so on), the risk status of such subgroups can be inferred from the data.

a) Persons characterized as being in the lower socio-economic strata have long been assigned high risk status with regard to mental illness.

(1) Bruce and Barbara Dohrenwend in an extensive review of the epidemiology of mental illness[11] found a consistent relationship between the lowest social strata and highest impairment rates and between highest social strata and lowest impairment rates in fifteen different community surveys.

(2) Another study conducted by Srole and his co-investigators in New York[12] provides similar data as shown in Table 1.

TABLE 1

Mental Impairment Category	Highest Socio-Economic Status Group	Lowest Socio-Economic Status Group
Well	30.0%	4.6%
Mild to moderate impairment	57.5%	48.1%
Severe impairment	12.5%	47.3%

(3) A much more recent study than any of those cited previously continues to demonstrate the

same finding (Table 2). These data were collected in New Haven, Connecticut by Myers and his co-workers in the study cited previously.

TABLE 2

Mental Impairment Category	Highest Social Class	Lowest Social Class
Low Symptom	40%	29%
Moderate Symptom	48%	46%
High Symptom	12%	25%

(4) This often-replicated association between mental illness and low socio-economic status identifies an important target group for both treatment and preventive efforts. Such a group deserves a high priority when it comes to resource allocation not only because of its high risk status but because the personal resources of group members place them in the poorest position economically to obtain needed services independently.

(5) If, indeed, persons in the lower socio-economic groups are at higher than normal risk, programs should be selectively directed at them. Clinics or at least satellites should be located in depressed areas. The availability of services must be made widely known in such areas. Good liaison must be established with other community agencies who serve the poor so that ready access to mental health treatment programs is assured. These would include general medical facilities, local clergymen, welfare workers and so on.

b) Another group often identified to be at high risk are the elderly.

(1) The Srole study cited previously and two of the major epidemiological studies by Leighton and co-workers[13] and Tischler and co-workers[14] have demonstrated an increasing prevalence of mental impairment with age (Table 3).

TABLE 3

Age Group	Srole	% Impaired Leighton	Tischler
20-29	15.3	7.4	3.5
30-39	23.2	18.6	14.2
40-49	23.2	22.3	14.2
50-59	30.8	23.0	16.4
60+	-	24.1	16.4

(2) A number of obvious contributing factors to this increased risk status can be cited. The elderly must confront illness, retirement, the diminution of sexual potency, personal loss and so on making their exposure to stress more frequent and more extreme.

(3) A stress not often highlighted which bears more careful consideration has been discussed by Kasl[15]. He points out that the elderly are both more sensitive and more vulnerable to forced moves which take them away from familiar surroundings. He has documented a deterioration of both physical and mental health as a consequence of such moves. Moreover, he has demonstrated that this risk can be overcome with enough preparation and support.

(4) The elderly are as ill-prepared economically to cope with mental illness as are the lower socio-economic groups cited previously and hence also can lay claim to a priority when it comes to resource allocation.

(5) Access to the elderly can be obtained by mental health centers through old age homes, activity centers for the elderly and so on. By making the elderly very aware of available treatment resources the chances of early treatment are maximized. In addition to this, preventive programs must be developed so that other community agencies which serve the elderly develop greater cognizance of their

mental health needs. This can prevent the occurrence of some difficulties or at least minimize them (e.g., the forced move situation).

9. A third approach to the study of high risk status comes from clinical research studies which either begin with a specific psychopathological state and look for the antecedent precipitants for it or start with some very specific event and look for the development of subsequent psychopathology. Such studies have focused not on general populations but on patient populations or on a specific population which has experienced some particular stressful event.

 a) A number of investigators have assigned a high risk status to children who have experienced a disrupted family life either as a consequence of divorce, extended parental absence or the death of a parent.

  (1) Using a retrospective study design Brown[16] observed that 41% of 216 depressed patients had lost one or more parents through death before the age of 15. This was much higher than the incidence of parental loss in the general population (12%) or in a general medical clinic population (19%).

  (2) Beck and his co-workers [17] examined 297 patients clinically using the Beck Depression Inventory in order to diagnose depression. Each patient was also questioned about parental loss. The results of this enquiry are summarized in Table 4.

TABLE 4

	% who lost at least one parent before age of 16	
	Severe Depression	Non-Depressed
Beck Depression Inventory	27.0	12.0
Clinical Examination	36.4	15.2

(3) Brill and co-workers[18] did not find an association between parental death and emotional disorder but did find an association between parental loss from all other causes and such disorders.

(4) Greer[19] compared suicide attempts with controls, looking for an association with the loss of a parent before the age of 15. Suicide attempts demonstrate a significantly higher rate of parental loss.

(5) In a now classic study, the Gluecks[20] compared delinquents and non-delinquents and found that 60% of the delinquents and only 34% of the non-delinquents came from broken homes. This disruption of family life occurred before age five twice as frequently in delinquents than in non-delinquents.

(6) Gregory[21] reviewed all existing studies in this area done before 1958. His review concludes that there is a demonstrable association between parental loss and the development of an antisocial personality or a psychoneurosis.

(7) The results of all of the above studies must be accepted with caution. All are retrospective. Definitions of what constitutes psychiatric disorder vary. Samples used are not always representative and comparisons are sometimes made between unlike groups.

(8) Despite all of the above, the association between disrupted family life and some form of later psychopathology has been replicated over and over. While the association does not demonstrate an etiological link it can serve at least to identify this high risk population as such.

(9) If we can identify such a high risk population early in life, we can attempt early intervention which hopefully can prevent the occurrence of psychopathology later in life.

(10) Attention can be focused on such children through the school setting, through pediatricians

and family practitioners, through children's clubs and so on.

b) Much of the original interest and work on the precipitation of psychopathology emanates from work on death and bereavement.

(1) Lindeman's[22] work on the impact upon survivors and surviving relatives of a Boston nightclub fire is one of the earliest expressions of interest in high risk groups.

(2) Since that time many investigators, including Elizabeth Kubler-Ross[23], have concluded that both the dying and their families and loved ones constitute a highly stressed group, and even more importantly that appropriate interventions can prevent the development of severe psychopathological states.

(3) Crisis services can be focused on victims and survivors through hospital, emergency medical facilities and through family physicians.

(4) Some investigators such as Silverman[24] have recommended a self-help approach which, for instance, mobilizes widows to assist other widows in weathering the grieving process.

c) A look at just a few of the many studies which have examined the impact of natural or man-made disasters[25, 26, 27, 28, 29] on whole populations ought to convince even the most skeptical that such victims constitute another high risk group.

(1) Such studies have demonstrated an increase in overall mortality rates from somatic illness as well as an increase in morbidity rates from somatic illness.

(2) These studies have also shown an increase in psychopathology and a sharp increment in the utilization of mental health treatment resources. Inpatient admission rates increase and outpatient facilities see a great influx of patients.

(3) Some investigators have argued that easy access to crisis intervention facilities is as

important as access to food, clothing, shelter and medical care for physical trauma in a disaster situation if such sequelae are to be reduced or prevented. Crisis clinics could easily be set up next to first aid stations or soup kitchens.

d) One of the most intriguing notions about high risk status to come along has been that propounded by Brenner[30] in a recent monograph.

(1) Brenner has examined short- and long-term economic cycles and has related these to state hospital admission rates. He has concluded from data subjected to sophisticated econometric techniques that the health of the economy can be correlated with increasing and decreasing admissions when there are controls for other possible factors.

(2) Brenner suggests that economic recession may be a powerful contributing precipitant of psychopathological states.

(3) Brenner's data base which comes from state hospital systems bears close scrutiny. His work deserves the replication that he is now attempting in a community treatment system but it should remind the reader of what has already been noted about the high risk status of low socio-economic groups.

(4) Unemployment and economic recession are societal problems that are far beyond the capacity of any mental health treatment program to solve directly. Such programs should, however, direct their early interventions at the appropriate high risk group. If the unemployed are indeed one such group, readily accessible and identifiable sources of help should be made available to them. Conceivably a mental health center could make the availability of its services known through the local unemployment insurance office or through the personnel office of an employer who is about to lay off a significant part of its work force.

e) Severe physical illness or injury associated or unassociated with hospitalization has long been associated with high risk status as regards mental illness.[31, 32, 33, 34]

(1) Depression, psychosis, anxiety states, phobias, work and sexual inhibitions have all been associated with serious medical illness and with major surgical procedures.

(2) All too often, intensive attention is paid to the medical or surgical condition but its psychological impact upon the individual goes unnoted and untreated. This frequently hampers the recovery process and may even lead to a circumstance where the patient is medically sound but psychologically crippled and nonfunctional. The depressed and anxiety-ridden patient whose myocardial infarction has healed but who cannot function at work or at home is a perfect example of this phenomenon. The woman who has just had a mastectomy for carcinoma of the breast but whose depression goes unnoted is another example.

(3) Mental health programs must focus educational efforts on physicians who currently do not utilize mental health professionals frequently enough in such cases.

(4) One surgical condition that has had an especially notable association with subsequent psychiatric disorder is hysterectomy. Barker[35] reports that 7% of 729 women who had a hysterectomy had subsequent psychiatric referral and that 80% of these referrals occurred within two years of the procedure. He found this to be 2. 5 times the rate after cholecystectomy and three times higher than the rate in a similar age group within the general population. The most common presenting symptom was depression. It is quite possible that other women also suffered from psychological symptoms but did not seek out help (7% may be the tip of the iceberg). Certainly, consideration must be given to the idea of offering a prehysterectomy psychological intervention to women who require this surgical procedure.

f) If injury which is the product of trauma creates high risk status, so too does injury, physical and psychological, that is the product of assault. Within the category of assault one of the potentially most injurious causes is undoubtedly rape.

(1) This cause of high risk status has gained increasing attention, so much so that special support for rape crisis facilities and for research was written into recent federal mental health legislation.

(2) In a recent study, Wolbert and Holmstrom[36] describe two phases which they suggest characterize the clinical course of the rape victim.

(a) A phase of acute disorganization in which anxiety, sadness, physical symptoms and in some cases a facade of calm and control are noted; and

(b) A reorganization phase in which nightmares and phobias are common.

(3) These investigators recommend a crisis intervention approach in which issue-oriented counseling and supportive measures are utilized. They suggest that in some cases more definitive long-term treatment will be necessary.

(4) Every emergency room which handles rape victims should have a crisis intervention facility available. Such a facility should be on the premises or readily accessible nearby by arrangement with some other facility.

g) Even ubiquitous events like moving to a new home or a new community have been linked to high risk status. Hall[37] has presented evidence that suggests that moving can produce intense enough stress in some individuals to precipitate psychopathological symptoms. Hence information about local mental health facilities ought to be included in the kind of material that is prepared for distribution to newcomers by organizations such as the Chamber of Commerce and the Welcome Wagon. More ambitious distribution schemes might work with and through public utilities and the telephone company.

h) The last of the high risk groups which we will consider here relates to another common life event, childbirth. A number of studies have suggested that childbirth is associated with high risk status for mental illness.

(1) One retrospective study by Jacobson and colleagues[38] examined a random sample of 467 recently delivered women and reported psychiatric symptom patterns after delivery (Table 5).

TABLE 5

# of Psychiatric Symptoms	% Reporting
0	17.8
1-3	36.2
4-6	19.8

Unfortunately they made no comparisons with the general population. They also noted that the onset of symptoms prior to or during pregnancy portends a poor course afterward.

(2) Another retrospective study in an Ohio community by Paffernbarger[39] reported the epidemiological findings in Table 6.

TABLE 6

Prepartum Mental Illness	5 per 10,000 population
Postpartum Mental Illness	19 per 10,000 population

Note the fourfold increase that this author reports. Rates were higher for older mothers and for mothers with prior history of mental illness either associated or not associated with a prior pregnancy.

(3) Pugh and his associates[40] observed much higher first admission rates than were expected to Massachusetts state hospitals among women in the 15-44 year age group.

(4) An obvious high risk woman is one who has borne a stillborn child or an abnormal child or who has suffered some sequelae of pregnancy.

(5) The above data warrant several steps:

(a) The education of family practitioners and obstetricians so that they will be appropriately alert to the possibility of postpartum psychopathology and can take early and definitive action.

(b) The education of pregnant women so that they are aware that emotional distress sometimes follows childbirth and that sources of help are available to them should this occur. Prevention efforts can focus on educating couples prior to delivery about childbirth and baby care.

(c) Education of hospital personnel, especially nursing personnel on obstetrical services, so they too will recognize such problems early.

(d) The establishment of appropriate crisis and other treatment facilities for women who wish to seek out treatment for postpartum distress.

10. Knowing specifically who is at higher than normal risk for mental illness can influence both the nature of the mental health programs mounted and the details of their implementation. The following questions and answers will illustrate this:

a) What kinds of programs should a community mental health center implement? A center located in a retirement area will focus more effort on developing programs for the elderly than will a center in a community of young married couples. The latter might focus on the problems related to pregnancy and parental loss, for instance. A center located in a large urban setting might develop a specialized rape crisis clinic while a rural center might not see enough rape victims to justify this specialization. In other words, the emphasis that a center places on particular programs will depend upon its general knowledge about high risk groups coupled with its specific knowledge about the nature of the community it serves.

b) Where should a center locate its services? High risk groups sometimes cluster geographically, and local knowledge or census data can identify such clusters. Particular areas may be plagued by high unemployment while other areas may have socioeconomically deprived groups, many old people and so on. Knowledge about high risk groups in general coupled with specific knowledge about <u>where</u> such groups cluster geographically can enable a center to locate clinics or satellites or to concentrate educational campaigns to achieve maximum impact.

c) How do we reach out to high risk groups? Obviously knowledge about who is at high risk gives important clues about this. Children can be reached through their schools, through recreational programs and through pediatricians and family physicians. The elderly can be reached through activity centers set up specifically for them but also through convalescent facilities. Clergymen with congregations in economically deprived areas can serve as an entry point for this group as can welfare workers. Centers must exercise ingenuity to tap all of the possible entry points and they must develop good working relationships with a variety of other agencies and professionals in order to be able to implement their ingenuity. The whole process starts, however, with a knowledge of <u>who one wishes to reach.</u>

11. Once one has identified high risk groups, what should be done next? The answer to this question must be divided into those programs which should be directed toward the high risk groups themselves[41, 42] and those programs which should be directed at social gatekeepers.

a) Several approaches to high risk groups themselves must be considered:

(1) To alert persons in high risk groups to the early signs and symptoms of emotional illness so that they can seek out early treatment when necessary (e.g., sadness, crying spells, a

loss of appetite and insomnia are signs of depression for which treatment is available).

(2) To suggest preventive measures which can be taken to reduce or minimize risk to patients or their families. For example, pregnancy can be a time of great stress and anxiety. An increased sense of coping capacity with a concomitant reduction of anxiety can often be achieved by taking a course on childbirth and baby care for expectant parents.

(3) To make persons in high risk groups aware of available sources of assistance for unmanageable stress and for frank symptoms of illness (e.g., a crisis clinic is located at such and such a place and is open 24 hours a day every day. Its staff helps all kinds of persons to sort out and get a handle on a wide variety of seemingly unmanageable situations).

b) Gatekeepers are important because they frequently have contact with high risk groups long before the community mental health program does. A wide variety of gatekeepers can be cited. These include the family physician, the local clergyman, a welfare worker, the local police and a whole range of others cited in the chapter on mental health education and public information.

(1) Gatekeepers should be alerted to the early signs and symptoms of mental illness. Early treatment can often improve prognosis but it can only be achieved if gatekeepers who see patients first know what to look for and who to look closely at. Gatekeepers will be more likely to identify early difficulties if they know who is at higher than average risk (e.g., if a family doctor is aware of the high risk status of his convalescing coronary patient, he is less apt to miss the symptoms of depression or anxiety and can intervene earlier or call in a consultant).

(2) Gatekeepers should know what to do once they have identified early difficulties in a high risk group member. For example, a clergyman is

called to the house of parishioners who are grieving the death of a child. He is able to provide a supportive atmosphere in which they can verbalize feelings of sadness, anger and guilt. He helps the family to focus on some of the specific steps they will take to readjust to their loss. He is watchful of signs of frank psychiatric impairment and is prepared to make an appropriate referral to a mental health center.

(3) Gatekeepers should be made aware of specific steps that they can take to reduce or eliminate high risk status. For example, a nurse in charge of the night shift of a convalescent home for the elderly is made aware by a mental health consultant of the increased vulnerability to confusion and disorientation in this group. It is suggested that she provide selected patients with night lights in order to minimize disorientation if they should awaken in the middle of the night.

c) The crisis clinic plays a special role with respect to high risk groups. Data on high risk groups can suggest target groups for which crisis intervention facilities should be readily accessible.

(1) Crisis facilities should be located close to or in neighborhoods that are likely to yield the highest number of high risk individuals or individuals exposed to higher levels of stress.

(2) Crisis facilities should make the availability of their services known to other service providers such as hospital emergency facilities, family doctors, clergymen, welfare workers, police and so on.

(3) High risk groups should become the target of informational campaigns which tell them about the location and hours of crisis intervention facilities.

(4) Where patient volume dictates, crisis intervention clinics should set up special programs for particular high risk groups. For example,

an increasing number of crisis clinics have special programs for depressed and suicidal persons and for victims of rape.

d) Other community mental health program development should also rest on what we know about high risk groups.

(1) Community mental health programs should assess their communities to determine what high risk groups can be identified, how large they are and where within the community they are located. For example, areas in Florida and Arizona which are well known as retirement communities will have large clusters of older persons for which specific programs which deal with illness, retirement, loss and so on can be developed. Other communities with younger families in the childbearing years can focus on programs of childbirth and childbearing. Communities with pockets of high unemployment can focus some of their early intervention programs on such groups. Satellite crisis clinics could be established in such pocket areas.

(2) Some of the data needed to identify and measure high risk group prevalence are available through census data or from data provided by the Bureau of Labor Statistics.

(3) Information about groups not identifiable through such sources must be obtained by surveying community leaders, other community agencies or by actual community surveys.

(4) Table 7 illustrates the kinds of programs, both preventive and treatment-oriented, which can be developed once high risk populations have been identified.

(5) Table 7 provides a very compact and limited survey of the available data on high risk populations.

TABLE 7

Type of intervention	Timing of intervention: Proreactive-intervention before stress occurs	Reactive-intervention after stress has occurred
Interventions to prevent the occurrence of stressful events (environmental improvement)	Establishment of policies which maximize contact between parents and hospitalized children	Not applicable
Interventions to reduce the exposure of vulnerable individuals to stress (environmental manipulation)	A screening program which attempts to identify and weed out Peace Corps candidates who it is predicted will have a poor adjustment to Peace Corps life	Job reassignment or assistance where signs of an inability to cope with existing job stresses have begun to manifest themselves
Interventions to reduce the potentially harmful consequences of stress (strengthening coping capacity)	A training program to prepare pregnant women to better cope with the expectable stress and problems of childbirth and parenthood	Crisis intervention and the use of social network supports to assist a grieving widow to better cope with the stress of the death of a spouse

REFERENCES

1. Brown, G. and Birley, J. Crises and Life Changes and the Onset of Schizophrenia. J. Hlth. Social Behav. 9: 203-214, 1968.

2. Birley, J. and Brown, G. Crises and Life Changes Preceding the Onset or Relapse of Acute Schizophrenia: Clinical Aspects. Br. J. Psychiatr. 116:327-333, 1970.

3. Smith, W. Critical Life Events and Preventive Strategies in Mental Health. Arch. Gen. Psychiatr. 25:103-109, 1971.

4. Paykel, E.S. Life Stress and Psychiatric Disorder: Applications of the Clinical Approach. In Stressful Life Events. B.S. and B.P. Dohrenwend (Eds.) New York: John Wiley and Sons, 1974.

5. Dohrenwend, B.S. Life Events as Stressors: A Methodological Inquiry. J. Hlth. Social Behav. 14:167-175, 1973.

6. Myers, J., Lindenthal, J. and Pepper, M. Social Class, Life Events and Psychiatric Symptoms. In Stressful Life Events. B.P. and B.S. Dohrenwend (Eds.) New York: Wiley Interscience, 1974.

7. Holmes, T. and Rahe, R. The Social Readjustment Rating Scale. J. Psychosomat. Res. 11:213-218, 1967.

8. Rahe, R. and Holmes, T. A Model for Life Changes and Illness Research. Arch. Gen. Psychiatr 31:172-180, 1974.

9. Gersten, J., Langner, T., Eisenberg, J. and Orzeck, L. Child Behavior and Life Events: Undesirable Change or Change Per Se. In Stressful Life Events. B.S. and B.P. Dohrenwend (Eds.). New York: John Wiley and Sons, 1974.

10. Vinokur, A. and Selzer, M. Desirable versus Undesirable Life Events: Their Relationship to Stress and Mental Distress. J. Personal. Soc. Psychol. 32:329-337, 1975.

11. Dohrenwend, B.P. and Dohrenwend, B.S. Social Status and Psychological Disorder. New York: John Wiley and Sons, 1969.

12. Srole, L., Langner, T., Michael, S., Opler, M. and Rennie, T. Mental Health in the Metropolis. New York: McGraw Hill, 1962.

13. Leighton, D.C., Harding, J.S., Macklin, D.B., MacMillan, A.M. and Leighton, A.H. The Character of Danger. New York: Basic Books, 1963.

14. Tischler, G., Henisz, J., Myers, J. and Boswell, P. Utilization of Mental Health Services. Arch. Gen. Psychiatr. 32:411-415, 1975.

15. Kasl, S. Physical and Mental Health Effects of Involuntary Relocation and Institutionalization of the Elderly: A Review. _Am J. Pub. Hlth._ 62:377-384, 1972.

16. Brown, F. Depression and Childhood Bereavement. _J. Ment.Sci._ 107:754-777, 1961.

17. Beck, A., Seth, B. and Tuthill, R. Childhood Bereavement and Adult Depression. _Arch. Gen. Psychiatr._ 9: 295-302, 1963.

18. Brill, N. and Liston, E. Parental Loss in Adults with Emotional Disorders. _Arch. Gen. Psychiatr._ 14:307-314, 1966.

19. Greer, S. The Relationship Between Parental Loss and Attempted Suicide: An Control Study. _Br. J. Psychiatr._ 110:698-705, 1964.

20. Glueck, S. and Glueck, E. _Unraveling Juvenile Delinquency._ Boston: Harvard U. Press, 1950.

21. Gregory, I. Studies of Parental Deprivation in Psychiatric Patients. _Am. J. Psychiatr._ 115:432, 1958.

22. Lindemann, E. Symptomatology and Management of Acute Grief. _Am. J. Psychiatr._ 101:141-148, 1944.

23. Kubler-Ross, E. On Death and Dying. _JAMA_ 221:174-179, 1972.

24. Silverman, P. The Widow-to-Widow Program. _Mental Hygiene_ 53:333-337, 1969.

25. Baren, J. Crisis Intervention: The Ice Cream Parlor Disaster. In _Emergency and Disaster Management._ H. Parad, H. Resnick and L. Parad (Eds.) Bowie, Md.: Charles Press, Inc., 1976.

26. Weil, R.J. and Dunsworth, F.A. Psychiatric Aspects of Disaster: Some Experiences During the Springhill Mining Disaster. _Canad. Psychiatr. Assoc. J._ 3:11-17, 1958.

27. Bennet, G. Bristol Floods-1968: A Controlled Survey of Effects on Health of a Local Community Disaster. _Br. Med. J._ 3:454-458, 1970.

28. Lyons, H. Psychiatric Sequelae of the Belfast Riots. Br. J. Psychiatr. 118:265-273, 1971.

29. Cohen, R. Post Disaster Mobilization of a Crisis Intervention Team: The Manaqua Experience. In Emergency and Disaster Management. H. Parad, H. Resnick and L. Parad (Eds.). Bowie, Md.: Charles Press, Inc., 1976.

30. Brenner, Harvey, M. Mental Illness and the Economy. Cambridge: Harvard University Press, 1973.

31. Wishnie, H., Hackett, T. and Cassem, M. Psychological Hazards of Convalescence Following Myocardial Infarction. JAMA 215:1292-1296, 1971.

32. Kasl, S. and Cobb, S. Some Psychological Factors Associated with Illness Behavior and Selected Illnesses. J. Chron. Dis. 17:325-345, 1964.

33. Groog, S., Levine, S. and Lurie, Z. The Heart Patient and the Recovery Process. Soc. Sci. and Med. 2:111-164, 1968.

34. Jenkins, C. Components of the Coronary Prone Behavior Pattern. J. Chron. Dis. 19:599-609, 1966.

35. Barker, M. Psychiatric Illness after Hysterectomy. Br. Med. J. 2:91-95, 1968.

36. Wolbert, A. and Holmstrom, L. Rape Trauma Syndrome. Am. J. Psychiatr. 131:981-986, 1974.

37. Hall, P. Some Clinical Aspects of Moving House as an Apparent Precipitant of Psychiatric Symptoms. J. Psychosomat. Res. 10:59-70, 1966.

38. Jacobson, L., Kaij, L. and Nilsson, A. Postpartum Mental Disorders in an Unselected Sample: Frequency of Symptoms and Predisposing Factors. Br. Med. J. 1:1640-1643, 1965.

39. Paffenbarger, R. Epidemiological Aspects of Parapartum Mental Illness. Br. J. Prevent. and Soc. Med. 18:189-195, 1964.

40. Pugh, T., Jerath, B., Schmidt, W., Reed, R. Rates of Mental Disease Related to Childbearing. NEJM: 268:1224-1228, 1963.

41. Yarvis, R. Crisis Intervention as a First Line of Defense. Psychiatr. Ann. 5:195-197, 1975.

42. Langsley, D. and Yarvis, R. Crisis Intervention Prevents Hospitalization: Pilot Program to Service Project. In Emergency and Disaster Management. H. Parad, H. Resnick and L. Parad (Eds.). Bowie, Md.: Charles Press Inc., 1976.

CHAPTER 11

CITIZEN PARTICIPATION

Donald G. Langsley, M.D.

1. History of citizen participation. In the original 1963 Mental Health Act (the beginning of the CMHC model), there was no mention of community involvement or citizen participation. It was assumed that local government and professional groups would design and implement a plan for providing mental health services. Even the regulations later adopted by the Department of Health, Education and Welfare did not require citizen participation, nor did they state that an official advisory group from the community must be involved in CMHC planning and management. However, by the late 1960's, consumerism and civil rights had developed into major national movements, and their forces were to have major impact on the development of federal health policies.

   a) The Consumer Movement asserted (and later demanded) that the consumer should not only be protected against professional and business groups, but that consumers themselves should be given more power and authority over those groups from whom they purchase services or products. At the same time, the media began to publicize new developments in the health sciences, making patients more aware of treatments and "remedies" which were, or soon would be, available upon completion of testing. Consumers often perceived the prudent delay between discovery and application as reluctance on the part of "organized medicine" to accept new challenges to old methodologies. Indeed, medicine began to be viewed as part of the "establishment", a term signifying bureaucratic unresponsiveness to the public's desires and needs. Out of this context of civil challenges to authority and a society-wide declaration of personal rights, a new patient-physician relationship emerged. Instead of simply following the advice of their physicians, patients began to ask questions. They expressed, in an informed fashion, the desire to participate in decisions affecting their health care. In fact, physicians began to be questioned sharply about their competence, their treatment plans and the process through which health plans for individuals and entire communities are developed. Comprehensive health planning came to be a conjoint activity with consumers and providers sharing decision-making responsibilities. The large amounts of public money which began to flow into health care budgets added impetus to the trend toward conjoint planning and more citizen control.

b) The first major health-related initiative of the civil rights movement dealt with the interests of those citizens who are treated involuntarily and whose civil rights, therefore, are vulnerable to violation. There were also concerns about whether patients being treated in the voluntary sector had given informed consent to such treatment, and whether the consent they gave was truly informed. The judicial system preempted Congress as the initial adjudicator of health-related civil rights issues. Civil rights lawyers and the Mental Health Law Project lawyers, as well as government lawyers, were disinclined to follow the lengthy, difficult course of seeking legislative action. Instead, they went directly to the courts and secured landmark decisions within existing laws. These decisions resolved certain issues pertaining to the detention and treatment of patients in involuntary hospitals (if patients are hospitalized involuntarily, the courts held that it must be for treatment and not simply for custody). The courts also established standards for those health care areas which had not achieved a reasonable level of quality. In case after case, the term "informed consent" underwent judicial scrutiny until its definition and interpretations were refined and procedures for ensuring that patients are made aware of their civil rights were enacted. Laws were later passed to protect patients from treatments which may require special precautions (e.g., electroconvulsive therapy), including a provision that protects patients from such treatment being administered involuntarily without appropriate indication. Further laws mandated additional consultation when such treatments are suggested under involuntary circumstances. In some states, the conditions under which psychosurgery can be performed have been determined by the courts; and judges have even felt themselves required to rule on the appropriateness of various psychosurgery procedures. Having begun their major thrust into the mental health field less than two decades ago, lawyers and legislators have now penetrated virtually every area of medical practice, from the point of diagnosis to the most sensitive aspects of patient treatment. All of their efforts, of course, have been waged in the name of concern for the patient.

c) With encouragement from the National Institute of Mental Health, the community mental health movement began to be viewed as a cooperative and collaborative activity of citizens and professionals. CMHC advisory boards representing the patient population were first recommended by NIMH, and then required. That led to a push for citizen control of community mental health centers, culminating in the 1975 legislation _requiring_ new centers to incorporate under a _governing_ (not advisory) board of trustees serving community interests.

2. _Reasons for requiring citizen participation, and then citizen control_, included:

a) A desire for direct input from citizens regarding the specific needs of their community;

b) A perceived need to sensitize the CMHC staff and planners to problems unique to their local populations, especially minority and disadvantaged cultures, through board-level representation (catchment areas serving a predominantly bilingual or foreign immigrant population were seen as especially in need of indigenous interfacing at the board level);

c) A need to have the CMHC's services supported vocally by a citizen member of the population (such a person is often needed to inform the public about services available, and to interpret and endorse the program where "mental illness stigma" is a particular problem);

d) A desire to include citizens in the planning process so that their knowledge of community resources and needs would be taken into account during the development of action plans for service and change (this implies that a center can provide community social action as well as professional services, and that citizens are better informed than professional staff members as to social actions needed); and

e) The desirability of having citizens advocate and lobby for their CMHC at budgetary and evaluative hearings before legislative and executive branches of government.

3. But problems arose in some areas where citizens controlled the CMHC. A few of the most commonly shared problems were:

a) CMHC's with governing boards composed of citizens with little or no experience in managing a health care delivery system experienced a multitude of administrative problems and failures (nor had any orientation or training for their citizens been provided by centers).

b) Some board members carrying a personal bias and/or socio-political objective used their controlling board status as a power base from which to achieve personal goals. A frequently observed disappointment was the case of board members who were admittedly less interested in mental health services than in creating jobs for minority citizens, and whose actions as board members clearly compromised the center. Others insisted on the recruitment of minority directors and senior staff with less regard for competence than for minority status. The drift toward social action was a consequence of both the board members and some of the staff of these centers.

c) Because citizens were often amateurs in management and did not know how to utilize staff effectively, an adversary posture developed between the professional staff and board members in some centers. As an outgrowth of what was considered to be a mistrustful attitude, some citizen members began to demand separate staff for their boards and even undertook evaluation of professional services in a manner thought to be highly threatening by some of the professional staff. (The evaluation of professional competence has traditionally been considered a peer-review prerogative, and not within the competence of general citizen groups.)

d) Questions were raised about whether the citizens on the boards truly represented the population being served. In some cases they were middle-class business and professional people who were dedicated to the community, but who were adjudged to be unaware of the needs and attitudes of poor people and minority groups. Even when only a fraction of the board members were middle-class types as described above, questions were still raised by various subcultures or community groups about the representation of their particular points of view. Power struggles were not unusual.

e) Where CMHC's were operated by government or by existing institutions (such as community hospitals) there was reluctance to turn over control of government property and funds to a citizen group. Indeed, many government groups felt that it would be illegal to do so. Community hospital trustees who also were responsible for CMHC facilities and budgets were equally reluctant to abrogate their responsibilities.

4. More recent laws have required citizen boards to perform certain tasks, including:

   a) Establishing general policies for the center;
   b) Approving the budget and various expenditures of the center;

c) Approving and appointing the center's director and staff; and
d) Planning and defining the center's programs

5. Centers with highly visible problems were frequently publicized, giving rise to questions about the viability of the citizen control model. Cases held up as examples of citizen board failures were those in which indigenous workers "representing the community" took control of a center and "fired" the professional staff. Such events or variations of them took place at New York City's Lincoln Hospital CMHC, at the Temple University CMHC in Philadelphia, and at the New Jersey College of Medicine. Other areas had similar problems with struggles between community groups and citizen boards.

6. The most successfully managed CMHC's were shown to have certain operational and management approaches in common. Some frequently shared characteristics of these centers were:

   a) A participatory approach to planning and program implementation (which discouraged power struggles);

   b) A clearly defined set of program ideals and internal policies which were accepted by the community (instead of simple external accountability); and

   c) The presence of mutually supportive alliances between consumer and provider

7. More recent amendments to the 1975 federal CMHC legislation acknowledged the special problems of some centers, and reversed their requirement for governing boards when the local government or community agencies are operating CMHC's or wish to establish one.

REFERENCES

1. Ozarin, L. D. Community Mental Health: Does it Work? Review of the Evaluation Literature. In An Assessment of the Community Mental Health Movement. W. F. Barton and C. J. Sanborn (Eds.). Lexington, Mass.: D. C. Heath, 1977, pp. 117-151.

2. Panzetta, A. F. Community Mental Health: Myth and Reality. Philadelphia: Lea and Febiger, 1971.

3. Tischler, G. L. The Effects of Consumer Control on the Delivery of Services. Amer. J. Orthopsychiatry 41:501-505, 1971.

CHAPTER 12

MENTAL HEALTH PROGRAM EVALUATION

Richard M. Yarvis, M.D., M.P.H.

1. Program evaluation must be defined and distinguished from other kinds of research activity that may take place in a mental health setting:

   a) Program evaluation consists of a set of mechanisms which are designed to measure change in the status of a patient population, an agency, or a community group at which some mental health program intervention has been directed.

   b) A program evaluation effort is charged with determining the amount, quality and impact of program efforts directed at such groups by a specific program.

   c) Unlike clinical research efforts which focus on specific treatment techniques and their effectiveness, program evaluation examines the effectiveness and efficiency with which a particular program effort, which may use a variety of techniques, impacts upon a given population. The focus is on the program effort rather than on the specific techniques.

   d) For example, an investigation of the effectiveness of lithium carbonate in the treatment of mania is an example of clinical research. An investigation of the success with which a specific outpatient program in a particular mental health center is able to stabilize chronic psychotic patients using a range of treatment techniques is an example of program evaluation.

e) The end product of program evaluation is data in the form of various measurements which serve as indicators of the quantitative and qualitative accomplishments of the program being monitored.

2. It is necessary to specify how evaluation efforts relate to the other basic functional components of a mental health program:

a) Evaluation efforts relate to all of the implementation components. These include each of the therapeutic and preventive programs which the mental health center carries on. Assessments of such programs may be continuous or periodic and the relationship is one of monitoring.

b) Evaluation efforts also relate to the planning component of the mental health program. The data collected by monitoring therapeutic and preventive programs are utilized in the center's planning functions where decisions about program change and resource allocation are made. Four general categories of information can be made available to planners by evaluation efforts[1].

(1) Data relating to program adequacy - What proportion of total need is the program addressing?

(2) Data relating to program appropriateness - Are resources being allocated as planned? Are high risk and special target populations being reached? Are all geographic areas receiving appropriate levels of service?

(3) Data relating to program effectiveness - Are program efforts having impact on the problems of persons being served?

(4) Data relating to program efficiency - Are program efforts being carried out as efficiently as they can be?

c) A continual cycle of planning, implementation, evaluation, modified planning, new implementation, reevaluation and so on should be established to relate evaluation to planning and implementation.

d) Evaluation efforts serve to provide planners and implementers with data on the basis of which programs can be continued, modified or eliminated. Such efforts serve as a key element in the development and ongoing management of community mental health programs.

e) Evaluation efforts can also provide positive proof to government funding sources and to community groups that a mental health program is productive and is responsive to community needs. Since competition for funding is often fierce and since government and community groups are often skeptical of the worth of community mental health programs, such proof can be extremely important.

3. To examine program adequacy, a number of techniques can be employed. Such measurements are important because no mental health center has yet begun to meet all of the mental health needs of its community. Hence a discrepancy always exists between the needy population that has been served and that whose needs have gone as yet unmet. Programs can only plan and provide services to fill gaps if they are aware of them:

a) Program adequacy speaks to the question: What proportion of the total community need is the center meeting?

b) An indirect method for assessing program adequacy relies on the development of utilization rates. Utilization rates relate the number of persons served by a program to the size of the entire population.

(1) To derive an overall utilization rate, the number of different persons served by the program is divided by the total number of persons living in the community being served and the answer multiplied by 100. This provides a utilization rate in percent.

(2) Utilization rates have been discussed in Chapter 3. The most recent available national data

for mental health centers show an average overall utilization rate of 1.1%[2] among 261 federally funded community mental health centers.

(3) Once computed, the overall utilization rate can be contrasted with epidemiological estimates of overall community impairment. In Chapter 3 these were noted to range between 10% and 25%.

c) A more direct method for assessing program adequacy relies on the development of <u>penetration rates.</u> Penetration rates relate the number of persons served by a program to the size of that part of the total population that is impaired.

(1) To derive an overall penetration rate, the number of impaired persons living in the population must be determined either by a community screening survey or extrapolated from existing data.

(2) Then the number of persons served by the program is divided by the total number of impaired persons and the answer multiplied by 100. This provides a penetration rate in percent.

d) In Table 1, we have carried out both of these procedures for the persons served by three mental health centers during a one-year period[3].

TABLE 1

	Total Population	Overall Utilization Rate	Estimated Impaired Population	Overall Penetration Rate
North Center 1974-75	141,042	1.1%	24,763	6.1%
South Center 1974-75	145,351	1.3%	28,315	6.5%
East Center 1974-75	112,983	0.9%	19,878	4.8%

Note that these centers served between 1% and 2% of the total population during a year and between 4% and 6% of those in need of service.

e) Overall utilization rates can be used to fulfill a number of functions.

(1) Comparisons between programs are possible. In this way, standards for expectable program output can be developed and used to monitor program performance. Note the differences in Table 1 and remember that every one-tenth percent difference between any of the figures shown represents 100 patients seen for each 100,000 persons in the population.

(2) Comparisons within a single program at successive time points can be made. In this way, change from year to year may be measured. Concerted efforts at casefinding can be assessed for success or failure if measurements of utilization rates are made before, during and after the casefinding program is begun.

f) Overall penetration rates can be used to fulfill a number of functions.

(1) Penetration rates are not only more precise than utilization rates but measure the relationship between the need for services and the demand for them as well.

(2) The overall penetration rate can be used like utilization rates to make comparisons between programs and within programs over time.

g) Another approach to the measurement of program adequacy is one which relies on the measurement of the volume of service delivered to a given population rather than on the number of persons served.

(1) Table 2 demonstrates this approach using services delivered over a one-year period.

(2) Such data can be utilized to compare programs as is done in Table 2 or to compare a single program over time.

TABLE 2

	South Center 1974-75	Median Level For All Federally Funded Centers in U.S. - 1973[4]
Ambulatory visits per 1000 pop.	116.7	75.5
Inpatient days of care per 1000 pop.	17.0	39.3
Day-treatment days of care per 1000 pop.	18.2	25.2

(3) Those who use the service volume approach would note any increment in service volume as a sign of greater program adequacy.

4. In making comparisons between programs remember that the size of the staff, the relative proportions of time devoted to treatment and the magnitude of services rendered to noncommunity members must all be taken into account. Any of these parameters may significantly affect service volume.

5. To examine program appropriateness, several parameters bear scrutiny; such measurements are important because mental health services are often not utilized uniformly by different population groups and because some groups in the population are at higher risk than others:

a) Program appropriateness speaks to issues such as:

(1) The degree to which mental health programs have reached high risk or traditionally neglected population groups;

(2) The degree to which all geographic areas of the community have received adequate service; and

(3) The degree to which resources are being allocated as planned

b) The degree to which a mental health program serves traditionally neglected and/or high risk populations is certainly one measure of the appropriateness of its activities.

(1) Age has been implicated in terms of both neglect and risk status. In Chapter 3 risk was noted to increase with age in several studies. Both children and the elderly have frequently been neglected populations.

(2) To monitor services to different age groups, utilization or penetration rates in Table 3 have been calculated in the same way as overall utilization and penetration rates but separately for each age group.

TABLE 3

South Center 1974-75[5]

Age Group	Utilization Rate in %	Penetration Rate in %
0-19	0.8	0.9
20-29	3.3	21.5
30-39	2.0	8.8
40-49	1.1	4.5
50-59	0.8	2.6
60+	0.4	1.7

(3) Note that the distributions for the utilization and penetration rates parallel each other quite closely. Note also that this center provided proportionately more service to young adults and less to children and the elderly during the year under scrutiny. These findings correspond quite closely with available national data.

(4) Remember that utilization rates standardize for differences in population composition so that service to different age groups can be compared directly. Remember also that penetration rates measure the relationship between need for services and demand for them.

(5) Active efforts to expand services to children and the elderly can be monitored by comparing utilization and/or penetration rates in successive years.

(6) Marital status was also implicated with respect to high risk status in Chapter 3. Note in Table 4 the high utilization and penetration rates for the divorced and separated group.

TABLE 4

South Center 1974-75[6]

	Utilization Rate in %	Penetration Rate in %
Married	0.8	3.5
Never Married	3.1	13.2
Separated and Divorced	6.7	16.1
Widowed	0.8	2.8

(7) The frequent neglect of minorities in the provision of mental health services requires attention to their utilization rates as presented in Table 5. Note the high utilization by blacks on the one hand and the low utilization by persons with a Spanish surname on the other. Attempts to rectify the latter can be monitored by comparing utilization rates in successive years.

TABLE 5

South Center 1974-75[7]

Racial/Ethnic Group	Utilization Rate in %
Caucasian	1.3
Black	2.1
Spanish Surname	0.6
All Other	0.5

(8) Finally, poverty has been implicated in risk status by a number of studies (see Chapter 3). Moreover, poor persons have traditionally had less access to mental health services than have more affluent groups. Note the inverse relationship between income and service utilization in Table 6. Clearly this center has actively served poor people.

TABLE 6

South Center 1974-75[8]

Income Level	Utilization Rate in %
0- 4,999	6.4
$ 5,000- 9,999	2.0
$10,000-14,999	0.6
$15,000+	0.3

(9) Utilization and penetration rates can be used to provide data to funding sources and to community groups when questions about the adequacy of services arise. An example will illustrate this use best. Example: A state governmental agency that oversees support to local mental health programs suspects that poor persons are failing to receive a fair share of the services being provided by the South Center's program. They requested some demonstration of the center chief's contention that this was not the case. The center chief supplied the data in the form of Table 6 which shows more than a twenty-fold difference in utilization between the highest and lowest income levels.

c) The degree of service rendered to different geographic areas of the community is another important measure of the appropriateness of a mental health program's activities.

(1) The catchment area is the most common geographic entity used to define a community for which a mental health center bears responsibility. It is a geographically contiguous area

which usually encompasses a population of 100,000 to 150,000 persons.

(2) All catchment areas are in turn subdivided into smaller geographic units. The most commonly employed subdivision is the census tract, a geographic entity containing 5,000 to 10,000 persons for which a variety of demographic, social and economic data are available.

(3) Overall utilization rates in percent can be calculated for each census tract within a catchment area by dividing the number of different persons seen by the population of the tract multiplied by 100. Such rates can then be compared between tracts, and tracts receiving low levels of service can be identified. In this way, areas of a community that are being neglected by a mental health program can be identified and appropriate corrective action taken.

(4) Using selected demographic, social and/or economic data available for census tracts, high priority census tracts can be identified. Social indicators such as median income, median years of education, percentage of minorities or children or the elderly have all been utilized to identify high priority tracts. These can then be monitored for utilization, and corrective action can be taken as necessary.

d) Monitoring resource allocation can also serve as an important measure of mental health center program appropriateness.

(1) Each center must decide for itself what the best balance for its activities is, based upon the emerging needs of its own community. Once this has been established and a program plan worked out, measurements of how staff time is being invested can be made. Sometimes such measurements of time investment in different activities reflect the center's plan and sometimes they reflect deviation from that process. Where the latter is true, managers can investigate and instigate change.

Without measurements of how time is being used, planning cannot be monitored and deviations from planning cannot be discovered.

(2) Another way to look at the appropriateness of resource allocation is to compare a center's performance with the performance levels of other comparable work settings. Small or moderate differences can be expected between centers but large discrepancies deserve scrutiny. Comparisons between the South Area Mental Health Center and a large group of federally funded CMHC's are provided in Table 7.

TABLE 7

Type of Activity	% of Total Time-South Area Mental Health Center: 4 Time Surveys 1974-75	Median % of Total Time: 323 Federally Funded Community Mental Health Centers, U.S. 1973[a]
Crisis Clinic (Emergency Care)	5.10	3.08
Inpatient	14.87	17.32
Day Treatment (Partial Care)	5.21	10.03
Outpatient	21.79	24.55
Management-Administration	16.35	N.A.
Research and Evaluation	3.04	1.33
Training (Inservice Training)	21.53	4.33
Community Service (Extramural Consultation)	11.85	5.18[b]

[a] Source: 1973 NIMH Profile for Federally Funded Community Mental Health Centers. See references.

[b] Excludes information dissemination and public education.

(3) While a center may use such comparative data to monitor its own program, it would be a mistake to place too much reliance on such comparisons. More important are a center's assessment of the particular needs of its own catchment area and the translation of those needs into priorities and resource allocation decisions.

6. To examine program effectiveness, a number of alternative measurement strategies must be considered. These alternatives include variations in study design and variations with respect to the endpoint which will be examined to determine outcome:

a) Three basic types of studies are commonly utilized in outcome- or effectiveness-oriented program evaluation[9].

(1) Archival studies: These are retrospective studies of record archives which can provide some conclusions about treatment outcome. No attempt at followup beyond the period covered by the treatment record is made.

(2) Retrospective followup studies: These too are retrospective studies but ones in which new followup data are obtained from patients no longer in treatment. From this data, conclusions are drawn about treatment effectiveness.

(3) Prospective outcome studies: In such studies patients are identified at the outset of treatment, and baseline measurements are made. At some interval after treatment, a new set of measurements is made so that pre- and post-treatment comparisons can be made.

b) Archival studies are most useful in examining the patterns of care rather than its actual outcome.

(1) Clinical records are difficult to use in assessing patient change since their content is variable and their appraisals of change lack standardization.

(2) Examinations of the patterns of care can be just as important as measurements of change.

In Table 8, some data are presented which illustrate the use of the archival approach to explore the relationship between diagnosis and the kind of ambulatory care received.[10]

TABLE 8

Type of Ambulatory Visit	Psychotic Patients	Neurotic Patients	Statistical Significance at the .05 Level
Crisis Clinic	3.7	0.7	Yes
Individual Psychotherapy	9.3	7.1	No
Group Psychotherapy	5.0	2.5	No
Conjoint/Family Therapy	0.8	0.3	No
Medication Clinic	7.3	0.5	Yes
Total Ambulatory Care	24.5	11.1	Yes

(3) Critics of community mental health have been quick to suggest that psychotic patients are given short shrift by centers. These kinds of archival data can resolve such issues.

c) The retrospective followup study permits some appraisal of outcome but no direct measurement of patient change.

(1) Patients can be contacted at some post-treatment interval and asked to rate the impact that treatment has had on them. The response, however, has no objective status and may reflect the patient's wish for improvement (or worsening for that matter) rather than real change.

(2) The retrospective followup study approach is best suited to inquiries about "client satisfaction." In essence this is simply a measure of consumer satisfaction with services rendered by a community mental health setting. No pretreatment data are needed to make such an assessment. "Client satisfaction" measures have come into vogue in recent times given the current climate of consumerism.

d) The prospective outcome study is actually more sophisticated and more patient-change-measurement oriented than either of the two previously discussed types.

(1) Pre-treatment baseline measurements are made which can later be compared with end-of-treatment and followup measurements.

(2) Both patients and therapists can be asked to assess patient status pre- and post-treatment.

(3) Standardized measurements can be made pre- and post-treatment. A number of approaches to this have become popular.

 (a) The use of assessment scales such as the General Well-Being Scale[11] or the MSIS Symptom Checklist[12] which measures symptom status and affective status (e.g., anxiety level).

 (b) The use of goal attainment scaling[13] in which patients and/or therapists enumerate treatment goals at the outset of treatment and later assess the degree to which these have been attained.

 (c) The use of social adjustment scales[14] which measure interpersonal, social and occupational functional status at appropriate intervals.

(4) Prospective outcome studies provide the best means by which to document patient change over the course of treatment. Moreover, they can be used to link patient change (improvement, no change, worsening) to particular patient groups (i.e., what kinds of patients improve, remain unchanged, or worsen with which kinds of treatment). Ultimately, data from such studies should enable us to match patients and treatment modalities in ways which will maximize improvement.

(5) Several cautions must be noted, however.

 (a) The measurement scales currently in use are less than perfect and will bear improvement over time. It is not always clear what they are measuring or how sensitively they measure it.

(b) Patient cooperation varies in community mental health settings. At times this contributes to high levels of missing data. Prospective studies in which multiple measures must be made over time are most affected by this.

7. Another approach to examining the quality of care rests on some assessment of the quality of clinical care. One way that such accountability can be satisfied involves the "peer review process."[5]

   a) Peer review is a term which refers to the process wherein ongoing treatment is evaluated by "peers", that is, professionals of comparable background. Its development has been stimulated by both federal legislation mandating the formation of Professional Standards Review Organizations (PSRO's) and the increasing emphasis on accountability by communities. The term "peer review" has been used to include:

      (1) Utilization review - authorization of ongoing treatment based on a judgment of the need for that service. It may also refer to claims review or a review of the claims to determine the need for a service after it has been rendered.

      (2) Quality assurance - focusing on the quality of care to be sure that the treatment was of appropriate quality and type. It uses agreed-upon criteria of "acceptable" treatment which have been developed by practicing professionals.

   b) The peer review process seeks to keep professionals involved in the determination of what is appropriate mental health practice.

   c) Peer review functions can be carried on by groups or committees. Their organization will vary from community to community but they are usually involved with several tasks:

      (1) Participation in the utilization review process

      (2) Developing standards for the quality of treatment and participating in quality assurance determinations

(3) Identifying the continuing education needs of the professionals who render care in the community

8. Program efficiency is the last of the evaluation parameters that we will consider. Efficiency studies encompass a range of issues that all relate to the facility with which available staff time is utilized:

a) One overall indicator of efficiency that can be measured would compare the total available staff time on the one hand and that proportion of it that eventuates in recorded program activity on the other.

(1) Such data can be obtained by periodic time surveys wherein each staff member records in detail his program activities for a specific period (e.g., one week).

(2) Using an expected work day of eight hours as a reference standard, time survey data can be used to examine efficiency as can be seen in the data presented in Table 9.16

TABLE 9

Time Survey	Total "Ideal" Available Staff Hours (Total Staff Days* X 8 Hours)	Total Actual Hours of Activity Recorded by the Time Surveys	Actual Hours as a % of "Ideal" Available Hours (Actual Hours ÷ "Ideal" Hours)
#1	238 X 8 = 1904 hours	1820 hours	95.6%
#2	302 X 8 = 2416 hours	2303 hours	95.3%
#3	320 X 8 = 2560 hours	2363 hours	92.3%
#4	282 X 8 = 2256 hours	1987 hours	88.1%
Total	1142 x 8 = 9136 hours	8473 hours	92.7%

* Actual days worked by staff during time survey.

(3) Efficiency ratios as presented in Table 9 can be compared between programs or within a given program at appropriate time intervals.

b) Another approach to the efficiency issue utilizes comparisons between expected time expenditures for given amounts of service and actual time expenditures for the same amount of service. This approach is illustrated in Table 10.

(1) By using the data in Table 10, center managers can know just "how expensive" each type of visit really is. Such knowledge should influence the direction a program takes and where its emphases lie, within the bounds of good clinical practice.

(2) The planning process will be facilitated whenever center managers can accurately predict what manpower resources will be needed to meet the expected demand for treatment services. With such data, managers should be able to allocate a definite proportion of total available clinical staff time to treatment services and know what will likely be left over for other activities.

(3) Table 10 provides a program manager an opportunity to compare his predictions of time requirements to provide service with actual experience. This leads either to the abandonment of one or more planning assumptions as unrealistic or inaccurate or to the administrative and/or clinical overhaul of program elements that are not being operated efficiently enough.

TABLE 10

Type of Outpatient Visit	Number of Visits (From Time Surveys*)	Predicted Hours per Visit (Developed Empirically)	Predicted Number of Hours	Actual Number of Hours Expended (From Time Surveys*)	Ratio of Actual to Predicted Hours
Individual	926	1.0 (1 hour ÷ 1 patient x 1 therapist)	926.0	922.25	0.99 (1% less time than expected)
Family/ Conjoint	82	1.5 (1.5 hours ÷ 1 family x 1 therapist)	123.0	146.75	1.19 (1.9% more time than expected)
Group	169	0.5 (1.5 hours ÷ 6 patients x 2 therapists)	84.5	99.25	1.17 (17% more time than expected)
Medication	375	0.5 (0.25 hours ÷ 1 patient x 2 therapists)	187.5	170.25	0.91 (9% less time than expected)
All Types of Visits			1321.0	1338.5	1.01 (1% more time than expected)

* Source: 4 quarterly time surveys.

REFERENCES

1. Denniston, D., Rosenstock, I. and Getting, V. Evaluation of Program Effectiveness. Publ. Hlth. Rep. 83: 323-335, 1968.

2. Profile of Community Mental Health Centers - 1973. Washington, D.C.: NIMH, 1975.

3. Yarvis, R., Edwards, D. and Langsley, D. Techniques for Assessment in Community Mental Health: Their Application to Planning and Program Management. Unpublished Manuscript, 1976.

4. National Institute of Mental Health - Division of Biometry and Epidemiology. Statistical Note #126, 1973.

5. Yarvis, R., et al. Above.

6. Yarvis, R., et al. Above.

7. Yarvis, R., et al. Above.

8. Yarvis, R., et al. Above.

9. Suchman, E. Evaluative Research. N.Y.: Russell Sage Foundation, 1967.

10. Yarvis, R., et al. Above.

11. Durpuy, H.J. Utility of the National Center for Health Statistics General Well-Being Schedule. Paper presented in the National Conference on Evaluation in Alcohol, Drug Abuse and Mental Health Programs. Washington, D.C., NIMH, 1974.

12. Laska, E.M. and Bank, R. Safeguarding Psychiatric Privacy: Computer Systems and their Uses. N.Y.: Wiley, 1975.

13. Kiresuk, T. and Sherman, R. Goal Attainment Scaling: A General Method for Evaluating Community Mental Health Programs. Comm. Ment. Hlth. J. 4:443-453, 1968.

14. Paykel, E. Dimensions of Social Adjustment in Depressed Women. J. Nerv. and Ment. Dis. 152:158-172, 1971.

15. American Psychiatric Association - Peer Review Committee. Manual of Peer Review. American Psychiatric Association. Washington, D.C., 1976.

16. Yarvis, R., et al. Above.

17. Yarvis, R., et al. Above.

CHAPTER 13

LEGISLATIVE ISSUES

Irving N. Berlin, M. D.

1. Needed revisions of the present community mental health act:

    a) Reduction of catchment areas:

        (1) Present catchment area boundaries, although they include between 75,000 and 125,000 people, usually end up at the maximum of 125,000 people with a staff that has been seriously reduced by the attrition of federal funds. Catchment areas should be redesigned to take in natural geographic areas which have to do primarily with a neighborhood containing at least an elementary and a junior high school and sometimes a high school with catchment areas of 100,000 and under.

        (2) Catchment areas of over 100,000 in ghettos or in densely populated areas have a concentration of acute mental health problems, usually adult and adolescent problems, so that the staff of the mental health center is overwhelmed with acute problems and cannot attend

to problems of children which are less obvious, although sometimes no less acute. Mental health centers in these catchment areas find it impossible to:

(a) Develop community liaison with other agencies,

(1) Especially to care for the geriatric population and to arrange programs for the elderly;

(2) Collaborate with schools, courts and other agencies on the behalf of children and adolescents since there is no time except for acute services; and

(3) Become involved in any preventive services or in any education and consultative services, which are important if the catchment area population is to become educated in the use of mental health services and learn to use mental health services at the earliest signs of stress and problems in adaptation rather than when suicide or psychosis forces the use of mental health facilities

b) All community mental health centers must be supported by staffing grants which are continuous.

(1) With very few exceptions, if any, the states have not picked up the declining federal balances in staffing patterns and therefore in many states where there is poor support for mental health the mental health centers have slowly, by virtue of the declining federal balance, suffered continuous attrition of staff until they are unable to carry out their mandate under the federal legislation.

c) There must be mandated services to children and the elderly.

(1) According to their numbers in the population, these mandated services must clearly be financially earmarked in proportion to the population to be served, and the monies that are allocated to the mental health center must clearly be spent on these services alone. If the mental health center is unable to mount these services, the mental health center must not be allocated the monies that are specifically appropriated for mandated services to children and the elderly.

(a) Specially trained personnel should be hired for children and geriatric services.

d) Group homes for the severely mentally ill of various ages, that is, the elderly, adults, adolescents and children, must be funded and staffed and controlled by the community mental health center in lieu of state hospitalization to alleviate the current congregation of severely mentally ill persons in towns and cities adjacent to closed state mental hospitals.

e) Each mental health center must have a clear plan for evaluating its services and its use of various therapeutic modalities. These evaluation programs must be federally financed through federal legislation, and evaluation plans must receive the approval of the regional National Institute of Mental Health (NIMH) office before the mental health center can operate.

2. <u>State legislation for community mental health centers:</u>

a) Each state must have an assessment of the mental health needs of the various regions of its state and have some plans for financing those needs beyond the federally legislated community mental health center staffing grants.

b) In most states, the federal staffing grants are minimal grants and provide a skeleton staff of professional and paraprofessional personnel for the treatment of the most acute mental disorders in the community.

(1) <u>Community outreach services:</u> States must, therefore, be encouraged by the federal

government to present plans which indicate support for community outreach services. Trained mental health outreach workers need to go into homes to provide a wide variety of support services to the acutely mentally ill and those who are single, elderly or mentally ill and living by themselves and unlikely, without aid, to come in for service. These services are necessary also for families where there are children with acute mental illness and where the family is unable to come in for service because there are other young children.

(2) Home treatment implementation: These community mental health aides must be in sufficient number to permit them to enter the home after a treatment plan has been worked out at the community mental health center and to help the family to implement such plans through involvement with the family in management of the acute or chronically ill adult, adolescent, child or elderly patient.

(3) Rehabilitative services: States must also provide for rehabilitative services which utilize local resources for employment training for those acute and chronically mentally ill who are sufficiently recovered and in remission so that they can begin to be trained for various private or public works programs.

(4) Integration with Health and Human Services (H. H. S.) agencies. States must also be able to show the federal government that they are capable of integrating their system of education, welfare and public health with the community mental health system to provide integrative services in education, and in welfare support to the mentally ill of all ages. This will enhance their capacity to function in society by being able to carry out the necessary programs to overcome educational deficits of many of the children, adolescents and adults which have resulted from their mental illness and thus prepare them for more meaningful roles in their community. The welfare system must indicate a willingness to employ

welfare workers with sufficient training or to provide sufficient training to their welfare employees so that they can use their contacts with welfare recipients to enhance the mental health of their clients.

(a) This includes being able to help their clients to deal with the welfare system when they are confused or irrational; and

(b) To be able to understand and react to the mentally ill person in such a way as to help him feel the concern and continued support of someone in the welfare system to reduce his sense of total isolation and confusion. Welfare workers must also be trained to make diagnoses of acute illness or exacerbation of illness in their clients so that referral to the mental health centers, or at least collaboration with those who are working with their clients in the mental health centers, can occur. There must also be clear agreement by the states that their public health facilities will provide adequate medical care and medical supervision to those severely disturbed or elderly disturbed patients who are homebound.

3. <u>Required new additions to the community mental health federal legislation</u>:

a) There must be special grants which allot specific amounts of money to children's services in each of the community mental health centers. These services must be specified, as must the specialized training of the staff, so that the omission or deletion of specific services or staffing components will result in the reduction of the grant by the amount allotted for such service. The minimum services to be financially supported from the federal grants are:

(1) Outpatient treatment of emotionally disturbed children using a variety of therapies:

(a) Group therapy, activity groups for small children and interactional and project group therapy for older children and adolescents.

(b) Family therapy as well as individual therapy must also be available. The law must specify the professional cadre that is to be permitted to work with children. This becomes especially important because in many mental health centers the professionals and paraprofessionals who work with a few of the children as time permits have had no special training in child development or in child psychopathology or child therapy and, therefore, are not particularly helpful to very disturbed children and their families.

(2) There must be outreach services into the community with efforts to identify mental illness and stress through early casefinding and consultation to preschools, head start and elementary schools. Thus, very severe behavior disturbances and psychoses of childhood as well as an incipient acting out and delinquent behavior which can be identified by the elementary school must be a primary target for outreach services in the community. There must be workers trained to work with children in therapy and to provide the variety of therapeutic interventions required which must include working with parents.

(3) There must be a specified liaison between the children's services of the community mental health center, the schools in the area, the protective services of the welfare department and those of the juvenile courts.

(a) There should be an adequate number of well trained workers in children's fields so that some may be attached on site to those schools which have the largest number of severely disturbed children.

(1) This might permit brief services to families and to children, as well as consultation with school personnel; and

(2) The diagnosis and disposition of those children who require more extended and intensive services which cannot be delivered on the school site.

(b) Consultation with the courts by the children's services division of the community mental health center must be mandated in order to produce a collaboration on behalf of children who are in custody or in foster placement because of child abuse or child neglect.

(1) These disturbed children will then receive adequate treatment through the community mental health centers;

(2) Well-supervised foster placement which will protect the child and permit his continued development; and

(3) There will be the initiation of a treatment process for the parents of the abused child

(c) The issues of custody and foster placement must also be dealt with by the community mental health center in collaboration with the welfare department's Aid to Dependent Children or the other units of the welfare department which deal with the neglected, abused child and foster care.

(4) Legislation to obligate the community mental health center and financial aid to develop liaison with mental health sanction-givers in minority communities and to collaborate with these and the indigenous healers, clergy, etc. in each community. The funding must permit:

(a) Consultation with clergy, curanderos, herbalists, and the shamen usually turned to by the indigenous population for help with mental health problems.

(b) Consultation with these indigenous practitioners to help them learn to diagnose and treat the mentally ill using in addition to their own remedies some of the insights gained from the mental health centers and being able to call upon the mental health centers to take care of those individuals whom they feel they are unable to treat and therefore must return such patients to them.

b) Services to the elderly:

(1) Federal legislation must support group living for those elderly who are mentally ill. This would establish a home base to reduce the disorientation which occurs with most elderly and, most acutely, with those who are both mentally ill and elderly and who have experienced frequent moves. Such efforts would reduce the continued agitation and inability to function in the community of many mentally ill elderly. It would reduce the need for both state hospital and nursing home care.

(2) The use of therapeutic groups on a daily basis to reduce the isolation and estrangement of the elderly, especially those with severe depression or psychosis.

(3) Medication necessary for the elderly to reduce their mental illness must be part of the planned allocations to the mental health centers.

(4) There must be planned use of the elderly who are mentally ill as they begin to recover to feel socially useful and important.

(a) Utilize the elderly in support of children's programs that are being carried out by the community mental health centers, such as day hospitals, programs for the retarded and other grandparent programs which utilize the skills of the elderly and continue to make them an important and useful part of the community.

(5) There need to be outreach programs and outreach workers,each assigned to specific elderly individuals who are mentally ill ,to be their advocate and liaison within the community and the mental health center. These individuals will facilitate problem-solving for the elderly and prevent commitment to hospitals or the resulting deterioration and terminal placement in nursing homes.

(a) It becomes important that there be one person in the mental health center or agency who is the advocate for the elderly person who is mentally ill.

4. Federal legislation must mandate center-based early intervention and prevention programs in the community.

a) There must be infant stimulation and parenting programs:

(1) These programs would be designed to identify high-risk infants and their mothers and through the use of stimulation programs reduce the possibility of their becoming mentally ill and developmentally disabled.

(2) The mothers in these programs must be involved in individual and group counseling to reduce their depression and mental illness and to make it possible for them to continue the infant stimulation in their home programs.

(a) There must, therefore, be outreach workers who can help mothers who are depressed and emotionally disturbed to carry out these programs within the home setting.

(b) Infants and small children identified by the public health well-child clinics with any specific problems, especially those of beginning autism or severe withdrawal or hyperactivity, those with severe feeding and allergic problems, and those whose mothers appear depressed or mentally ill, must have a resource for referral, such as an infant stimulation and parenting program preferably related to a community mental health program so that treatment to mothers may be initiated if necessary.

(3) Any infants and small children with chronic illnesses uncovered in infancy, preschool or head start must have the opportunity for early intervention and treatment in the children's service of the mental health center along with the prescribed medical treatment and the necessary parenting and early stimulation programming.

c) Preschool:

(1) There must be early identification of problems in development and severe behavior in the preschool child. Work with these children usually in groups and counseling with parents primarily in groups would reduce the amount of severe disturbance which interferes with learning and with family living. Severe disturbances may begin to alienate the child and parent to the degree that many parents abandon their children or neglect and abuse them.

(2) There must be a parenting program for parents who have difficulties with their preschool children.

(a) Counseling should be available for those parents who are severely disturbed or depressed.

(b) There must be opportunities for the parents to learn to work with their children through parenting classes.

(c) Opportunities must be made for the parents to learn to become teachers of their children and involved in their children's educational process in the classroom and at home as a way of enhancing the mental health of the child who becomes aware of the parents' concern and interest in his or her education.

(3) In the preschools, early recognition of child abuse and neglect must occur with referral to the necessary authorities in the welfare and judicial systems.

(a) The mental health system should be available for developmental assessment and treatment programs as required.

(b) Child and parent programs to help abusing parents to parent their child should be developed.

(c) Individual treatment must be provided for the severely abused and neglected and psychologically traumatized child to reverse the emotional disturbance which is the result of the abuse and neglect.

c) The school-age child: Severe learning and behavior problems of the school-age child can be identified so that they will not become chronic problems if they are identified in the elementary schools. Developmental problems and neurological deficits must also be identified:

(1) Children with a variety of developmental handicaps with severe emotional problems must be helped as well as their parents in and through group work with children and group counseling with their parents.

d) Early intervention and prevention must also occur with the adolescent age group. Early recognition of depression and alterations in school behavior which are often preludes to psychosis and suicide may provide early intervention. Mental health workers and school counselors must be trained to work with the depressed and withdrawn adolescent who is usually also having learning problems and problems in communication and is thus difficult to work with. Training should be given in work with the adolescent and the family regarding issues of strivings for independence and autonomy to help reduce the conflicts in the families which may lead to acute decompensation of the adolescent or to suicide.

(1) Work-study programs such as a peer counseling program or others which enable adolescents to feel useful because they are learning skills which can be used in helping them to think about what kinds of jobs or professions they may enjoy and be good at would be extremely important for the mental health of the adolescent.

e) Young parents programs: From the prenatal visits in the public health clinics to the postnatal public health clinic visits, it becomes clear that young parents who have not yet learned about parenting need instruction.

(1) Some of these parents are sufficiently emotionally disturbed to require, in addition, counseling from the mental health center; and

(2) Instruction in parenting often needs to be oriented both to the developmental needs of the child and the particular troubles and developmental deficits of the parents.

(3) Mental health personnel need to be involved with pediatricians and public health personnel to help them to identify the vulnerable parents who are likely to have difficulty in parenting and who might become the dissatisfied, disgruntled and abusing parents in this society.

(4) Help to parents through diagnosis and treatment planning where children have severe psychological illnesses needs to be provided:

(a) Clear evaluation of the services available and help in obtaining them;

(b) Professional help necessary to do good developmental and psycho-social evaluations of the illness;

(c) Trained professionals to recognize the obstacles in parents to hear and understand the diagnosis with a recognition of the need to repeat interpretations and clarify before a treatment plan is evolved;

(d) Subsidized training of all mental health professionals and paraprofessionals to become effective in diagnosis, its interpretation and planning for treatment; and

(e) Special training in treatment techniques with child and parents

f) Size of the problem: About 3% of the child population requiring mental health services is a clearly gross underestimate in terms of the kinds of malfunctioning seen in the school situation. The following are two examples of ways in which present budgetary issues might be dealt with:

(1) The Office of Child Development head start program in its parent-child program now has sufficient research background to indicate that it is possible to extend these programs downward to age one and to provide enrichment programs for both the infant and small child and mothers which might greatly enhance the capacity of both the child and the mother in their own development, one as a young child and the other as the more effective parent. In addition, those young parents who have learned to become effective infant and young mother teachers can be developed into high quality paraprofessionals who will greatly extend the services possible.

(2) Another example of the need to integrate services occurs when one looks at the Bureau of Maternal and Child Health and its need for increased funding to deal with such important issues as the sudden infant death syndrome,

the hemophiliac syndrome, the crippled children's and maternal and child health programs which are funded through the state. Many of these deal with specific disease entities like sickle cell anemia, Tay Sachs disease, cystic fibrosis, hemophilia, muscular dystrophy, etc.

(a) However, in none of these programs is it also mandated that sick children be assessed developmentally so that one can predict in terms of their past development what their needs are to help them function more fully at the present and in the future rather than becoming simply chronically ill children who function at a minimum level.

(b) At the same time an assessment of the developmental issues within the family might help the mothers, especially to function more effectively with the diseased child, and to recognize the developmental needs of her other children and to obtain some help in dealing with both the diseased child and her normal children to optimize their development.

(c) The overriding principle previously mentioned is best illustrated here again when one looks at the fact that in the past in maternal and child health, the disease of the child is looked upon as an event, not a process to be considered in terms of its antecedent effects on the child and its prospective developmental effects upon the child which could be anticipated and worked with to maximize the child's capacity to function.

(d) Similarly, the disease and its impact upon the mother, the other parent and the siblings are also looked upon as a single event without recognizing that many mothers confronted by a chronically diseased child might be so depressed and so overwhelmed by other problems that they might not understand or be able to carry out the instructions given to them. Many mothers may not even be able to give the medication appropriately. Here too the event vs. the developmental process needs to be looked at carefully in terms of the family, mother and father and children, to optimize the development of the children and parents in terms of their future functioning.

g) Adult programs: Both industry and community alertness to beginning signs of depression, psychotic thinking and behavior and general reduction of adaptive functioning:

(1) Requires training of mental health professionals and paraprofessionals but mostly of health professionals most likely to see these adults and to be alert to these signs. They also need to learn how and where to make referrals.

(2) Community mental health centers, if given financial support, can provide such training to health professionals and become the back-up diagnostic and treatment resources as needed.

(a) Early recognition and treatment is critical to early return to adaptive functioning.

h) Programs for the elderly:

(1) Require training of health personnel, mostly nurses and aides, to get to know the elderly and become knowledgeable about the signs of stress and beginning decompensation.

(2) Communities, most homes for the aged and most nursing homes have no personnel to survey the elderly persons in their purview and pick out those whose adaptations are stressed and require immediate help to prevent hospital or other institutional care with its cost to the individual and society.

(3) Current knowledge indicates that the elderly can be greatly helped to maintain their effectiveness if they are given recognition and support during periods of stress.

(4) Programmatic use of retired persons in areas of community need must be provided so that vocational, professional and interpersonal skills are not wasted. A sense of continued usefulness to society and continued competence and effectiveness as a person are keys to such prevention and early intervention methods which must be federally supported.

CHAPTER 14

ISSUES FOR THE COMMUNITY MENTAL HEALTH MOVEMENT

Donald G. Langsley, M.D.

1. Basic purpose of the CMHC: Treatment of the mentally ill. In his 1963 message to the nation, President John F. Kennedy recommended the establishment of community mental health programs that would:

> ...bestow the full benefits of our society on those who suffer from mental disabilities ... provide for early diagnosis and continuous and comprehensive care, in the community of those suffering from these disorders ... stimulate improvements in the level of care given the mentally disabled in our State and private institutions, and to reorient those programs to a community-centered approach ... reduce, over a number of years, and by thousands, the persons confined to these institutions ... retain in and return to the community the mentally ill and mentally retarded, and there to restore and revitalize their lives through better health programs.

In commenting on the desirability of linking mental health with general health services, he said:

> Ideally, the Center could be located at an appropriate community general hospital, many of which already have psychiatric units. In such instances, additional services and facilities could be added, either all at once or in several stages, to fill out the comprehensive program.

As for therapists, Kennedy envisioned a program wherein:

> ...private physicians, including general practitioners, psychiatrists and other medical specialists, would all be able to participate directly and cooperatively in the work of the Center. For the first time, a large proportion of our private practitioners will have the opportunity to treat their patients in a mental health facility served by an auxiliary professional staff that is directly and quickly available for outpatient and inpatient care...

In addition to raising the subject of mental illness to unprecedented national attention, President Kennedy's message clearly emphasized the importance and advantages of treating mentally ill patients in the community. But the keystone of that plan was its base in the local hospital, where teams of mental health specialists could administer the new psychoactive drugs and psycho-social approaches, thus "for the first time", making it possible to treat large numbers of the mentally disordered on an outpatient basis. In the intervening years since that plan was adopted, however, CMHC's have drifted away from their original purpose (treatment of the mentally ill) and into a social service model (e.g., marital counseling and crisis intervention for predictable family problems). That drift has been accompanied by a transplantation of the CMHC's locus from community hospitals to community based or "store front" operations. Whereas they were initially sponsored by local hospitals or governments with community advisory boards, CMHC's have now been co-opted by community governance boards. A critical consequence of these events has been the wholesale neglect of our chronically mentally ill, especially the deinstitutionalized, and the apparent abandonment of medical leadership as reflected in the drop in psychiatric staffing of centers. Moreover, there has been considerable criticism of the more recent activation of CMHC's, indicating that this "bold new approach" is not working and that, in fact, the system has begun to crumble as a result of having lost its keystone, its sense of purpose and commitment. President Jimmy Carter appointed a President's Commission on Mental Health as one of his first acts in office following his inauguration in 1977; and his wife, Rosalynn Carter, was named the Honorary Chairperson of that commission. In 1978, the Commission concluded its report by suggesting a return to the original purpose of the CMHC: treatment of the mentally ill. The Commission's report also included several other recommendations and, more recently, its members have proposed a new law entitled the Mental Health Systems Act. As this book is being published, that proposed piece of legislation was passed by Congress in 1980, and it clearly has pointed the way toward remedying some of the problems associated with recent drifts in the community mental health movement.

2. Health or social service? The most commonly heard complaint about CMHC's focuses upon their orientation toward correcting social problems rather than treating the mentally ill. In keeping with their newfound orientation, services offered by many centers have been designed around reality problems such as poverty, vocational placement, child care, and direct social action. Though social services are an important adjunct to health care, they cannot be substituted for it. Those CMHC's which have given the seriously mentally ill a low priority and have shifted their attention instead to the problems of daily living have, ironically, become the perpetrators of unjust social ills by turning their backs on those most in need. In 1975, more than 20% of the patients seen by CMHC's were diagnosed as not mentally ill, and given labels such as "social maladjustment without manifest psychiatric disorder." Though most would agree that successful operation of a CMHC requires linkages with the social services located elsewhere in the community, there are indications that some centers have shifted away from a health base for the ulterior purpose of avoiding medical leadership. In such cases, there is often a philosophical undercurrent which would suggest that resolution of social problems can cure or prevent serious mental disorder. Whether or not funding for centers can more readily be obtained from social services or health resources, this fundamental issue of orientation impacts, more than any other, on the quality and future of the community mental health movement. It is one which must be faced and settled if we intend to carry out President Kennedy's initiative of moving the locus of treatment into the community, and if the CMHC is to become the major setting for the treatment of mental illness.

3. <u>Prevention.</u> Though one hope of the community mental health movement has always been to avoid mental illness through prevention, that hope has not been realized. Original planners of the community mental health movement anticipated that mental illness would diminish as social problems were addressed and solved, but that too has not been the case. Primary prevention can only be applied to mental illness when its "causes" are found, but with the exceptions of tertiary syphilis and the mental problems of pellagra, those causes have not appeared. Findings from work on early intervention with children hold some promise for reducing childhood mental problems, including learning and behavioral disorders, but such claims have not yet been firmly established. Prevention efforts at the CMHC level are probably of greatest value in secondary prevention, i.e., in early identification and prompt treatment in order to prevent chronicity. Even though there is an acknowledged lack of data supporting the effectiveness of primary prevention, its popularity has not been dampened. Basic research which may someday open the door to real prevention should not be deterred, but the fundamental role of the CMHC is not that of carrying on such research. Rather, the community mental health movement should encourage those institutions which do basic research on the causes of mental disorder (mainly universities) to expand their efforts to discover causes of mental disorder, and to find more effective prevention and treatment techniques. It has not been shown that mental disorder in adults can be prevented with lectures on child rearing or talks given at PTA's to parents of those future adults; and until such time as these methods yield conclusive prevention results, we should maintain our focus on proven techniques for actual treatment. For the present, secondary prevention offers more hope for circumventing mental illness since these activities have been demonstrated to interfere with regression, hospitalism and the consequences of unnecessary institutionalization.

4. <u>Neglect of the chronic patients.</u> The community mental health movement had hardly been launched before medical journals and the news media began publicizing the problems of deinstitutionalization. Many patients were discharged from mental hospitals before community programs were prepared to receive them. Some were ignored altogether, and remanded to a dire existence in crowded hotels or on the streets. CMHC's serving the institution's geographic area were not involved in treatment planning

before the patient was discharged. Programs and facilities for providing the rehabilitation required for this group were not in place. Maintenance medication programs wherein patients were only rarely seen by physicians were the extent of the care they found in the community. Supervised living arrangements which are a necessary part of community placement for such individuals were not functioning. Patients were not conscientiously tracked, and many of them "fell through the cracks." A number of exposés were published in various metropolitan areas revealing that "deinstitutionalization" had resulted in little more than disenfranchisement for those most sadly neglected. "Mental illness ghettos" developed in areas near state mental hospitals where patients had been discharged in wholesale fashion. Judicial decisions which mandated "least restrictive alternatives" for the mentally ill actually hastened the dislodging of many patients. A reform movement based on the high moral platform of humane treatment for the mentally ill had resulted in even more grievous conditions for many of those so "liberated." This apalling irony was not lost on journalistic observers. A New York Times editorial of April 8, 1974 (entitled "Civil Liberty for What?") asked rhetorically, "What kind of crusade is it to condemn sick and fearful people to shift for themselves in an often hostile world?" Before it can begin to add new goals and directions, the community mental health movement must first complete its original one, treating the mentally ill, and it must correct these deficiencies in its services to the most seriously ill. A high priority must therefore be given to the development of specialized services and facilities needed for this population, including:

a) Comprehensive emergency services with mobile teams for providing immediate consultation at residential settings, or for bringing patients to centers for crisis treatment;

b) Acute inpatient facilities for the seriously decompensated;

c) Subacute 24-hour treatment facilities in nongeneral hospital settings;

d) Partial hospitalization programs designed for chronic patients;

e) Outpatient programs, including aftercare-medication clinics for providing psychosocial therapy as well as drugs;

f) Supervised living arrangements where mental health staff are in contact with the residential home operators; and

g) Training programs for independent living (rehabilitation-resocialization), including therapeutic patient clubs, Community Friends, and interaction with community based paraprofessionals

Centers must remember their commitment to treating all of the mentally ill, chronic as well as acute patients. They should also emphasize certain programmatic aspects of their services if the health of their patients and the movement as a whole is to be decisively improved. Some of those programs are:

a) Aggressive and continuous patient follow-up, conducted with a true sense of responsibility on the part of the CMHC staff;

b) Public information-education programs to reduce mental illness stigma and acquaint the public with programs available at centers;

c) Program monitoring to evaluate services for chronic patients, and to assess their impact on short-term and long-term outcomes of such patients; and

d) Attendance to political realities, with the involvement of citizen groups as well as relatives of patients as needed in getting the CMHC message across to legislators, government executives and to the public at large

5. The underserved. A variety of groups of citizens are presently underserved by the CMHC's. Two immediate tasks of this movement should be the identification of these and other underserved groups, and the establishment of more effective treatment programs to meet their needs. These groups include:

a) Children are probably the most underserved of all groups, and yet they represent the most important and greatest asset of tomorrow's world. Although centers have expanded general outpatient treatment programs, their programmatic commitment to children is far below what should be indicated by the numbers of children they serve. Some centers have a showpiece program which is generally affiliated with a university, but this is not enough. Direct services for children must be increased, with an even greater increase in the number of CMHC child psychiatrists. Treatment for depressed mothers has been shown to influence the mental state of their children. Preschool programs and other work with schools have been demonstrated to reduce the number of dropouts who might otherwise have become involved in delinquency and drug abuse.

b) The aged are also seriously underserved. Many older citizens with behavioral problems are removed to nursing homes for what is considered to be "irreversible senility", when in fact, many of them are simply suffering from treatable depressions. At present, there are only a handful of psychiatrists skilled in the specialized treatment of the elderly, and the same shortage exists in all of the mental health professions. One explanation for this dilemma has to do with American society's characteristically negative attitudes toward the aged. Older patients are often difficult to treat because many of them cannot easily come to CMHC's or other treatment centers. Interest in this group of people is rising, however, and new programs are being developed. The most promising of these new programs are those which emphasize careful evaluation and treatments close to home which permit even the acutely ill to remain with their families.

c) Minority populations require specialized services designed to meet the individual needs of their cultures and languages. Because they are often socially and economically disadvantaged themselves, it is difficult to recruit minority staff who would naturally be sensitive to such needs. A strong commitment to affirmative action on the part of CMHC's is therefore needed. Minority representatives on the boards of such centers have too often demonstrated a primary focus on civil rights issues, particularly minority employment, and this has served to interfere with specific mental health services needed. Staff members who are not minority representatives can be helped to achieve some understanding and sensitivity if special training is offered in this area, but the need for affirmative action cannot be answered by such measures.

d) The physically ill are also being neglected by CMHC's. Various studies have shown that at least 10% of those seen in a community mental health center for "psychiatric symptoms" are relieved of those symptoms when their physical illness is recognized and treated. Patients who have both functional mental disorder and organic disease will improve when the physical illness is diagnosed and treated, just as those with physical illness improve when their psychiatric symptoms receive adequate treatment. Greater collaboration with primary care physicians is one of the challenges for the CMHC.

6. Staffing. The overall professional staff of CMHC's has grown over the past decade, but numbers of psychiatric and other medical personnel staff have been sharply reduced. In 1970, there were approximately seven psychiatrists in the average center, but by 1976, the number of psychiatrists per center had fallen to 4.3. Today, more than 50% of the centers have fewer than 2.3 psychiatrists, less than enough to assure quality treatment by any reasonable standards. In the same period of time during which psychiatric staff declined, the number of psychologists per center increased by more than 70%, and the number of social workers rose by nearly 30%. Nursing personnel have remained at about the same level of staffing. Those psychiatrists who do work in the centers are often part-time employees whose functions have been reduced to signing prescriptions. They do not have the time to participate regularly in treatment planning or to consult with other staff performing treatment. Reports from a large proportion of psychiatrists in such centers indicate a commonly shared lack of job satisfaction and lowered professional prestige as a result of their association with CMHC's. Many feel that physicians should be responsible for patient evaluation, diagnosis and treatment planning; and that they should be available throughout the treatment for consultation on problems which may arise. The physician should also be available for consultation and education of other medical and non-medical personnel in

non-center settings. Among reasons for the desirability of this more inclusive role are the interactions of psychological and biological components in any presenting patient. Psychiatrists have the medical and psychiatric training which equips them to be especially skillful in patient evaluation, management, and the education of non-psychiatric physicians who treat patients with all types of problems. Though it was once required that a physician be the clinical director of the CMHC, there has been a steady and rapid decline in the proportion of centers employing psychiatrists as directors, from 56% in 1973 to 22% in 1977. Because it has been shown conclusively that centers require a multidisciplinary staff, and that the quality of their services suffer when such imbalances as these occur, one of the most immediate problems confronting CMHC's will be the diminishing numbers and roles of their psychiatrists.

7. Effectiveness of treatment and preventive programs. As in all other settings where psychiatric and mental health programs exist, there is a paucity of "hard" data concerning the effectiveness of treatment for mental disorder. This criticism is more frequently leveled at psychotherapy than at other types of treatment (e.g., biological or pharmacological approaches). Recent Congressional statements have called for demonstrations of the efficacy and safety of psychotherapy before long-term commitments to federal third-party payment (National Health Insurance) for such treatment can be made. Some of the reasons for focusing on psychotherapy relate to the fact that there are between 120 and 140 different types of psychotherapy described in the literature. A recent review of 500 different studies measuring the outcome of psychotherapy indicates a trend in the direction of positive results. But although the overall trend is definitely positive, there are few, if any, studies which test specific kinds of psychotherapy for given types of mental disorder. Research in this area is needed to demonstrate the cost effectiveness of psychotherapy, and to convince its detractors that psychotherapy should be funded under national health insurance. Several have suggested that the cost of treating mental disorder is offset by concomitant decreases in the costs for other medical care, including hospitalization, laboratory tests and physician services. A recent survey of 25 different studies relating to this "offset" theory suggests that such a reduction in the cost of other medical services does occur, though the studies are not

methodologically perfect. In one study from Germany, 845 individuals who received intensive psychotherapy or psychoanalysis were followed for five years after treatment. Their use of general hospital services dropped from an average of 5.3 days per year to 0.8. This compares to an average hospital use rate of 2.5 days per year for the total insured group. Such an offsetting reduction in hospital costs, especially at today's high prices, would be convincing evidence of psychotherapy's cost effectiveness. Research data on the effectiveness of prevention techniques and/or mental health consultation are lacking. In general, the entire field of community mental health must face the need for more intensive program evaluation, thus to assure the public that these programs being funded by public monies are operated wisely, effectively and safely for those who receive treatment.

8. Governance issues. The original concept of community mental health was based upon the notion that the community should participate cooperatively with professionals in the establishment and governance of the CMHC. The initial legislation thus required that a community advisory board, representative of community populations, be included in every CMHC plan. The purposes of this requirement were to assure mutual planning; to enable the board to interpret the center's services to the community; to bring input from the community into the center's planning; and to encourage the board to become an advocate of its center. However, the NIMH later led to a recommendation for community control, rather than community participation. This approach was similar to others of the consumer movement which called for at least 51% consumer representation on health planning groups. Such twists in health planning reflected society's general movement toward mistrust of the "establishment", in this case, hospitals and other providers. Serious complications for CMHC's operated by local governments or institutions with their own boards (such as hospitals and universities) have been the result. Municipal governments which funded CMHC's were not anxious to turn over the responsibility of controlling government expenditures to citizen groups. Neither were the hospitals or universities which had established and operated CMHC's ready to turn over control of their physical facilities, programs, staffs and budgets to groups of citizens. Governments, universities and hospitals viewed themselves as being asked to surrender authority without being relieved of responsibility for CMHC

programs. The NIMH also contributed to this dilemma by approving more and more CMHC's with a community, rather than a hospital, base. These particular CMHC's were often subjected to control by part-time, untrained boards composed of citizens who were admittedly biased in several key areas, and who wished to see their own personal, societal agendas placed above the best interests of the CMHC and its patients. To many of the disadvantaged board members, this power represented an opportunity to rectify mistreatment they had suffered in the past; sometimes, this was carried out with prejudicial vengeance equal to that which they had known previously. Some inner-city boards were controlled by people whose main interest was in creating jobs for the poor, rather than in designing treatment programs for their patient populations. In the process, antiprofessional attitudes developed, and many of these board members began to believe that they could operate a center as effectively as professional groups, without their input or assistance. The socially-oriented posture of some boards made it even more difficult for CMHC's to obtain government funding. State governments were more eager to fund state mental health programs when they owned the institutions and employed the staff. To these legislators, CMHC's had become nongovernment citizen groups seeking government funds, and appropriations reflected that perception. CMHC's received a priority rating well below that of state owned and operated services. In its counterobservation that government, with its bureaucracy and civil service procedures, may be less efficient and less responsive to the needs of citizens, the President's Commission on Mental Health suggested that there be a return to the advisory board model when governments or other institutions operate the CMHC's.

9. Rational planning for mental health. Planning is for the purpose of making maximal use of existing resources so as to meet the prospective needs of a population. Participatory planning, that which includes providers, consumers and community planning representatives, is one of the hallmarks of community mental health. One of the issues for the community mental health movement, therefore, is the need to plan in a rational manner, rather than through the perfunctory armchair process which has often characterized such efforts. In order to make the process rational and to make best use of limited resources, resource allocation should be related to planning; and planning

should be a servo-mechanism through which continual review allows changes to be based on feedback about the success of previous plans. In this manner, planning will be linked to evaluation. In addition, planning should be a continuous process with annual review based on recent and new developments in the mental health field. Plans should strive for quantifiable and measurable objectives, and the mechanisms for achieving such objectives should include: (a) need assessments; (b) program evaluations; and (c) resource inventories... all of which lead to: (d) allocation of resources in a continuously updated plan.. followed by: (e) quantitative and qualitative monitoring of the plan's objectives. Further evaluation and outcome measures would then lead to subsequent planning and further change in this ongoing process.

10. Insurance coverage and funding problems. CMHC's are more likely to secure funding for their direct services; however, dependance upon governmental subsidies for these direct services, whether at the state or federal level, would be a mistake. The federal program was clearly meant to provide "start up" funds for the CMHC's five-year (later extended to eight-year) grants, after which time the CMHC's were to find their own funding. In recent years, Medicaid and Medicare have come to be sources of funding for CMHC's, with considerable variability among the states regarding their Medicaid programs. Services covered in such manner have been limited to direct treatment, usually that which is provided by, or supervised by, a physician. Insurance programs have become another source of funding, again for direct services, and again, usually limited to those services provided by, or supervised by, a physician. The several proposals for National Health Insurance have varied in the degree to which they would be willing to include mental health services. Generally, there have been limits on the mental health services to be covered. The deductibles under catastrophic insurance proposals have been so large that they eclipse the cost of the very limited mental health services allowed, thus excluding coverage of mental disorder under those catastrophic insurance plans. This will surely be one of the concerns of CMHC's if they intend to continue. Perhaps the National Health Insurance plan which will ultimately evolve will allow insurance plans, patient fees (limited because of the sliding scale) and government health plans to fund the CMHC's direct treatment services, with the government alone funding preventive and

consultative services offered by CMHC's. Third-party health plans generally define their responsibility as limited to direct treatment. Another factor that will determine funding will be the creation of a "single budget for mental health", instead of separate budgets for institutions (state hospitals) and community mental health centers. The divided-budget approach makes the two groups compete with one another, and it generally favors the institutions. A single budget approach, with local determination as to whether funds are spent in state hospitals or in the community, is the system which has made California's community mental health program so successful.

11. Low profile. If the CMHC is truly to serve the total population of its catchment area, it must adequately publicize the services and make them known to citizens and the agencies which offer social and health services. Unfortunately, not many centers have made such an adequate effort. This type of public information can be combined with campaigns to reduce the stigma of mental illness and to encourage early identification of problems which can benefit from prompt treatment. The CMHC should become a well-known community resource for the treatment of all citizens, rather than being viewed as a provider of second-class services for second-class citizens. If all community mental health centers would strive to achieve those ideals first envisioned by President Kennedy, their image, as well as the state of mental health in our nation, would be immeasurably enhanced.

REFERENCES

1. American Medical Association. Evaluation of Community Mental Health Centers: Report of an Advisory Panel of the Council on Scientific Affairs. Approved by House of Delegates. December, 1979. Chicago: AMA, 1979.

2. Bachrach, L. L. Deinstitutionalization: An Analytical Review and Sociological Perspective. Washington, D. C.: U. S. Govt. Printing Office, 1976.

3. Barton, W. and Sanborn, C. J. (Eds.). An Assessment of the Community Mental Health Movement. Lexington, Mass.: D. C. Heath, 1977.

4. Becker, A. and Schulberg, H. C. Phasing Out State Hospitals: A Psychiatric Dilemma. NEJM 294:255, 1976.

5. Beigel, A. and Levenson, A. I. (Eds.). The Community Mental Health Center. New York: Basic Books, 1972.

6. Borus, J. Issues Critical to the Survival of Community Mental Health. Am. J. Psychiatr. 135:1029, 1978.

7. DeMas, F. M. Medical, Nonmedical or Antimedical Models for Mental Health Centers. Am. J. Psychiatr. 133:875, 1974.

8. Kennedy, J. F. Message from the President of the United States to the 88th Congress. Document No. 58, February 5, 1963.

9. Lamb, H. R. and Goertzel, U. The Long-Term Patient in the Era of Community Treatment. Arch. Gen. Psychiatry 34:679, 1977.

10. Langsley, D. G. Community Psychiatry. Chapter 45.1. In Comprehensive Textbook of Psychiatry III. H. I. Kaplan, A. M. Freedman and B. J. Sadock (Eds.). Baltimore: Williams & Wilkins, 1980.

11. Langsley, D. G., Barter, J. T. and Yarvis, R. M.: Deinstitutionalization: The Sacramento Story. Comprehensive Psychiatry 19:479, 1978.

12. Panzetta, A. Community Mental Health: Myth and Reality. Philadelphia: Lea and Febiger, 1971.

13. President's Commission on Mental Health. Report to the President From the President's Commission on Mental Health, 4 volumes. U. S. Govt. Printing Office, 1978.

14. Winslow, W. W. The Changing Role of Psychiatrists in Community Mental Health Centers. Am. J. Psychiatr. 136:24, 1979.

INDEX